African Holistic Health for Women

Ancient Tribal Remedies, African American Herbalism, Black Medicine, and Other Ancestral Cures to Revive Your Divine Feminine Energy by Healing the Body and Soul

NYA LOVE

TALE OF CONTENTS

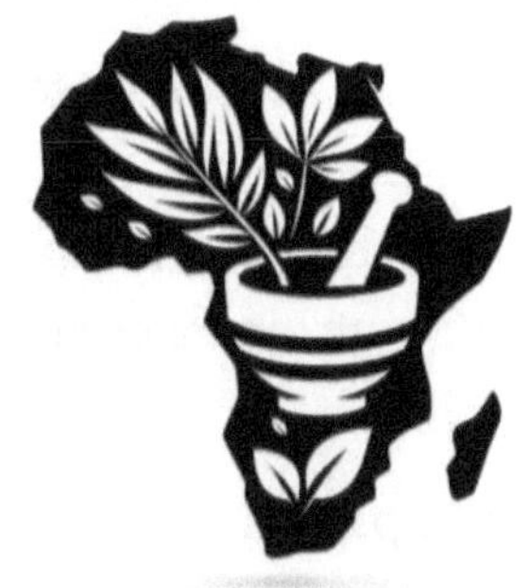

Introduction

Welcome to African Holistic Health for Women. In this book, we will embark on a transformative journey that celebrates the rich heritage of African holistic health practices specifically tailored for women.

Through the exploration of ancient tribal remedies and the wisdom of African American herbalism, we will delve into the depths of ancestral cures to revitalize your mind, body, and soul.

Are you ready to unlock the secrets to harnessing your divine feminine energy and embracing holistic healing in its purest form?

Well, let's begin with the basics. I would like to introduce a few definitions that will help you understand the main concepts of this book and know what to expect. You may be wondering, what exactly is holistic health? What do the concepts of healing and Divine Feminine energy—which are found everywhere in new age spiritual communities nowadays—really mean?

Holistic health is an approach that considers the whole person— encompassing physical, mental, emotional, and spiritual well-being. It recognizes the interconnectedness of these aspects and aims to achieve balance and harmony. Healing, within the context of holistic health, refers to the restoration of optimal health and well-being on all levels. It involves addressing the root causes of imbalances rather than merely treating symptoms.

Wholeness refers to a state of complete integration and unity. It involves nurturing all aspects of oneself and embracing the interconnectedness of mind, body, and spirit. Achieving wholeness requires self-awareness, self-care, and a commitment to personal growth and development.

By adopting a holistic approach to health, women can cultivate a sense of empowerment and take an active role in their well-being. This includes engaging in practices such as mindfulness, nutrition, exercise, stress management, and self-reflection. Embracing holistic health and striving for wholeness can lead to a more balanced, fulfilling, and vibrant life.

So, what does all this have to do with Divine Feminine energy?

Connecting with Divine Feminine energy nourishes women and empowers us in every area of our lives. Divine Feminine (DF) energy is the sacred and powerful creation energy that embodies qualities such as intuition, compassion, creativity, nurturing, and connection to the divine creative essence that permeates all of existence. The DF represents the feminine aspect of divinity, and she is often called upon when one needs to cultivate grace, wisdom, and emotional depth.

You can explore more on DF energy through my other book Goddess Energy: Liberate the Divine Feminine You Have Hidden.

By adopting a holistic approach to health, women can tap into the power of their own inner Divine Feminine energy and cultivate personal strength and empowered living.

Engaging in the practices explored in this book and striving for wholeness enables women to embrace their innate wisdom, intuition, and creativity, leading to a more balanced, fulfilling, and vibrant life. All of these are qualities of the Divine Feminine that bring women in harmony with the healed goddess within them.

Packed with both knowledge and tools for application, get ready to experience a life-changing voyage that honors the abundant legacy of African holistic health traditions. You will discover the ancient remedies passed down through ancestral lineages of women connected with the Divine Feminine within.

So, let's begin.

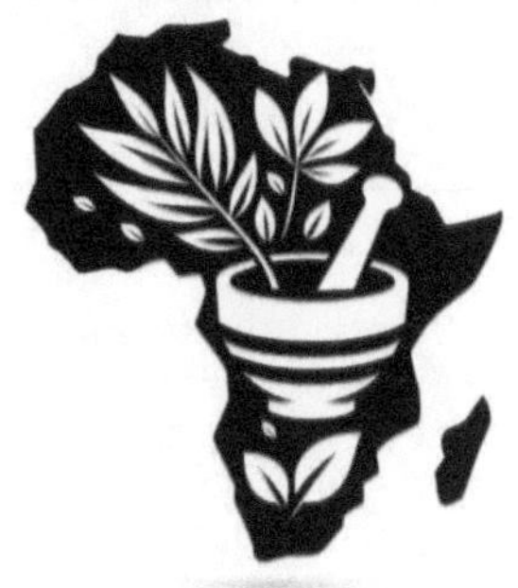

Chapter 1
Introduction to Ancient Tribal Remedies

Let us begin our captivating journey through time as we delve into the rich *herstory* and profound significance of ancient tribal remedies.

Our exploration takes us deep into the heart of diverse tribal healing practices, where we will unravel the intricate tapestry of cultural and spiritual aspects intertwined with ancestral remedies.

From the sacred rituals passed down through generations to the profound wisdom of indigenous healers, we will uncover the hidden gems of ancient traditions that continue to resonate in our modern world. Through this guidebook, we will unlock the secrets of these time-honored remedies and discover their enduring relevance in the tapestry of human well-being.

Tribal Health and Well-being

Have you ever wondered how some African American women stay so vibrant and seem to barely age? Well, when you nourish your body, mind, heart, and spirit, you can too.

Africa is home to a rich tapestry of diverse healing practices employed by different tribes. These tribes have developed traditional methods and techniques to promote health and well-being within their communities*. From herbal remedies to spiritual rituals, the healing practices across Africa vary greatly, reflecting the unique cultural and geographical contexts of each tribe.

In the Maasai tribe of East Africa, healing practices often revolve around the use of medicinal plants^. The Maasai have a deep knowledge of the local flora and utilize various herbs and roots to treat ailments. Their healers, known as Laibon, possess extensive knowledge of these plants and their healing properties*. Through their expertise, they are able to alleviate physical and spiritual ailments within the community.

Moving westward to the Yoruba tribe of Nigeria, we find a strong emphasis on spiritual healing practices. The Yoruba believe that illness is often caused by spiritual imbalances or malevolent forces*. Therefore, their healing methods involve connecting with the spiritual realm through divination, prayer, and rituals. Traditional healers, known as Babalawo or Iyanifa, serve as intermediaries between the physical and spiritual worlds, providing guidance and performing ceremonies to restore harmony and well-being*.

In Southern Africa, the San people developed unique healing practices deeply rooted in their hunter-gatherer lifestyle*. The San believed that illness is caused by disharmony between humans and nature*. To restore balance, their healers, known as shamans, sangomas, or medicine men, engaged in trance-like states induced by rhythmic dancing and chanting*. During these altered states of consciousness, they communicated with the spirit world and received guidance on how to heal the individual or the community.

The Himba tribe of Namibia practices a form of healing known as "hot stone therapy."* This ancient technique involves placing heated stones on specific points of the body to promote relaxation, relieve muscle tension, and stimulate blood circulation. The Himba believe that the stones possess healing energy that can restore balance and vitality, this is reflected in the concept of animism*.

The diverse range of healing practices used by different tribes across Africa showcases the deep connection between culture, spirituality, and well-being. From herbal remedies to spiritual rituals, each tribe has developed unique methods to address physical, emotional, and spiritual ailments within their communities. These healing practices not only provide relief but also serve as a testament to the rich cultural heritage and wisdom of African tribes.

With so much wisdom available, it can be difficult to know where to begin. The aim of this book is to make the process of cultivating holistic health as a woman easier for you as each chapter unfolds.

Let's explore a few of the techniques and tribal healing practices I have highlighted.

Herbalism

Tribal healing practices encompass a rich tapestry of traditions passed down through generations, These traditions offer unique insights into the power of nature, energy, and ritual. Among these practices, herbalism stands as a cornerstone.

Herbalism is an ancient practice that harnesses the healing power of plants to enhance both physical and spiritual well-being. It has been utilized by various cultures throughout history, each with their unique knowledge and traditions.

For example, the indigenous tribes residing in the lush Amazon rainforest have long relied on the medicinal properties of plants like ayahuasca and cat's claw to address a wide range of physical, psychological, and emotional ailments*.

These tribes have passed down their wisdom, recognizing the profound connection between nature and human health.

Ayahuasca, a sacred plant brew, is known for its transformative and visionary properties, often used in spiritual ceremonies to gain insight and healing*. Cat's claw, on the other hand, possesses anti-inflammatory and immune-boosting qualities, making it a valuable remedy for various health conditions*.

The rich biodiversity of the Amazon rainforest provides an abundant source of medicinal plants, each with its unique healing properties*. Herbalism, in any context, serves as a bridge between ancient wisdom and modern healthcare, offering alternative approaches to wellness that honor the power of nature.

By tapping into the vast potential of herbal remedies, women can explore holistic healing methods that promote balance and harmony within the body, mind, and spirit.

Energy Healing

Energy healing is another fascinating aspect of tribal healing practices. This approach also recognizes the interconnectedness of mind, body, and spirit, and seeks to restore balance and harmony within the individual. One example of energy healing is Reiki, a Japanese technique that channels universal life force energy to promote healing and relaxation.

Reiki is a gentle and non-invasive healing technique that promotes balance and harmony within the body, mind, and spirit. Through the use of light touch or hovering hands, a Reiki practitioner channels universal life force energy to the recipient, allowing it to flow freely and address any imbalances or blockages.

Energy healing is not just an Eastern or Western practice, However. African energy healing*

This holistic approach to healing aims to restore the body's natural ability to heal itself, promoting relaxation, stress reduction, and overall well-being. With its soothing and nurturing qualities, energy healing offers a unique and transformative experience that supports physical, emotional, and spiritual healing.

Tribal communities often have their own unique forms of energy healing, such as the Navajo concept of "Hózhǫ́ǫ́gíí *," which focuses on restoring harmony and balance. This ancient healing tradition relies on the power of prayer, song, and ceremonial practices to promote physical, emotional, and spiritual well-being.

Through the intricate weaving of rituals and sacred chants, the Navajo people believe they can tap into the natural energies of the universe, facilitating healing and rejuvenation. The practice of Hózhǫ́ǫ́gíí not only addresses the individual's ailments but also seeks to restore harmony within the community and the natural world*. It is a testament to the deep connection between tribal cultures and their profound understanding of the interplay between energy, spirituality, and healing.

Ceremonial Rituals

Ritual ceremonies play a vital role in tribal healing practices, serving as powerful conduits for spiritual connection and transformation. These ceremonies often involve sacred rituals, dances, and chants that facilitate healing on multiple levels. For instance, the sweat lodge ceremony, practiced by various Native American tribes, combines intense heat, steam, and prayer to purify the body, mind, and spirit*. This ceremony is believed to promote physical detoxification, emotional release, and spiritual renewal.

In exploring tribal healing practices, it is important to recognize that these traditions are deeply rooted in cultural and spiritual contexts. They are not merely alternative therapies, but holistic systems of healing that honor the interconnectedness of all beings and the natural world. By examining examples of herbalism, energy healing, and ritual ceremonies within tribal communities, we gain a profound appreciation for the wisdom and efficacy of these practices.

Through herbalism, energy healing, and ritual ceremonies, tribal communities have developed profound insights into the healing potential of nature, energy, and spiritual connection. These practices offer valuable lessons and inspiration for women seeking alternative approaches to health and well-being. We can foster a deeper understanding of ourselves, our connection to the natural world, and the power of healing that resides within us all.

Cultural and Spiritual Aspects of Ancestral Remedies

As you've probably noticed, ancestral remedies are deeply intertwined with the cultural and spiritual beliefs of the associated African tribes they stem from.

Understanding the cultural and spiritual aspects of ancestral remedies is crucial in comprehending their significance and contextualizing them as African American women. These remedies are intricately woven into the fabric of cultural and spiritual beliefs, forming an integral part of their community's identity and heritage.

The connection between ancestral remedies and African tribes goes beyond mere physical healing, it encompasses a profound spiritual connection to the ancestors and the natural world.

In African tribes, ancestral remedies are viewed as sacred and powerful tools that bridge the gap between the physical and spiritual realms*. They are believed to carry the wisdom and guidance of the ancestors, who are revered as guardians and protectors of the community*. The remedies are seen as a means of accessing ancestral knowledge and tapping into the collective wisdom of generations past.

Rituals and ceremonies play a significant role in the practice of ancestral remedies. These rituals are conducted with utmost respect and reverence, often led by spiritual leaders or healers who possess deep knowledge of the ancestral traditions*. The ceremonies serve as a way to honor the ancestors, seek their blessings, and establish a spiritual connection with them.

During these rituals, specific sacred traditions are followed to ensure the efficacy of the ancestral remedies. The process may involve the use of symbolic objects, such as herbs, animal parts, or sacred artifacts, which are believed to carry spiritual energy*. The healers perform intricate rituals, invoking the spirits of the ancestors and seeking their guidance in the healing process.

The ceremonies also serve as a communal gathering, bringing together the entire tribe to participate in the healing rituals. This collective involvement fosters a sense of unity, reinforcing the cultural and spiritual bonds within the community. It is a time for storytelling, sharing wisdom, and passing down ancestral knowledge to the younger generations.

The belief in ancestral remedies reflects how African tribes view health holistically, recognizing the interconnectedness of the body, mind, and spirit. Ancestral remedies are seen as a means of restoring balance and harmony within the individual and the community as a whole.

Understanding and appreciating these cultural and spiritual aspects is essential in recognizing the richness and depth of ancestral remedies in African tribal traditions.

The Role of Shamans and Elders in Preserving Ancestral Knowledge for Tribal Healing and Holistic Health

In many indigenous cultures around the world, the role of shamans, healers, sangomas, and elders is crucial in preserving and passing down ancestral knowledge for tribal healing and holistic health. These individuals possess deep wisdom, spiritual connection, and a profound understanding of the natural world. A number of these healers are often women. Let's take a look at the various kinds.

Shamans

Shamans are spiritual leaders who bridge the physical and spiritual realms*. They are believed to have the ability to communicate with spirits, ancestors, and the natural world. Shamans play a vital role in preserving ancestral knowledge by acting as intermediaries between the human and spirit realms.

They acquire knowledge through visions, dreams, and direct communication with spirits. Through rituals, ceremonies, and healing practices, shamans pass down this knowledge to future generations*. For example, they may use sacred plants, chants, and dances to heal physical, emotional, and spiritual ailments.

Healers

Healers are people who possess specialized knowledge and skills in traditional medicine and healing practices*. They work with herbs, plants, and natural remedies to restore balance and harmony within the body. Healers often learn their craft from their ancestors and undergo rigorous training and apprenticeships. They hold a deep understanding of the medicinal properties of plants, the body's energy systems, and the interplay between physical and spiritual health. By passing down their knowledge to apprentices, healers ensure the preservation of traditional healing practices.

A modern-day, more westernized example of a healer is a lightworker. Many healers today are women, this is in part because returning to wholeness and harmony is the realm of the Divine Feminine. It can be inspiring for a woman today to take the torch that has been passed down to her and lead as the light bearer for a more holistic world.

Sangomas

Sangomas, found primarily in Southern Africa, are traditional healers who play a vital role in tribal communities *. They are believed to have been chosen by their ancestors and possess the ability to communicate with the spirit world*. Sangomas undergo a rigorous initiation process, which includes training, rituals, and ceremonies. They are responsible for diagnosing and treating various ailments, including physical, mental, and spiritual imbalances*. Sangomas also serve as counselors, mediators, and spiritual guides within their communities, passing down their knowledge through oral traditions and apprenticeships.

Elders

Elders hold a revered position within African tribal communities. They are the custodians of ancestral knowledge and wisdom accumulated over generations. Elders possess a deep understanding of traditional healing practices, rituals, and cultural traditions. They serve as mentors, advisors, and storytellers, passing down their knowledge through oral traditions *.

Elders play a crucial role in preserving the cultural identity and holistic health practices of their communities. Their wisdom and guidance ensure the continuity of ancestral knowledge for future generations.

The role of shamans, healers, sangomas, and elders in preserving and passing down ancestral knowledge for tribal healing and holistic health is invaluable. Through their spiritual connection, specialized skills, and deep understanding of the natural world, these gifted people ensure the continuity of traditional healing practices. By bridging the gap between the physical and spiritual realms, they provide guidance, healing, and wisdom to their communities.

The preservation of ancestral knowledge is not only essential for tribal healing but also for the cultural identity and holistic well-being of indigenous communities worldwide.

Now let's briefly take a look at how these ancient traditions apply in modern times.

Modern Day Application of Ancient Traditions

Ancient traditions have always held a certain allure, captivating our imagination and connecting us to our roots. In modern times, the relevance of these age-old customs and practices is a topic of great interest and debate. One area that particularly stands out is the continued significance of ancient tribal remedies in the present day.

Tribal remedies have been used for centuries to address various ailments and promote overall well-being. Despite the advancements in modern medicine, these traditional remedies continue to hold a place of importance in many communities around the world.

One example of such a remedy is the use of herbal concoctions to treat common ailments. Ancient tribes have long relied on the healing properties of plants and herbs to alleviate symptoms and restore health

*. For instance, the use of chamomile tea to soothe digestive issues or lavender oil to promote relaxation and sleep are practices that have stood the test of time.

Moreover, the continued significance of ancient tribal remedies can also be attributed to their holistic approach to healing. Unlike modern medicine, which often focuses solely on treating symptoms, traditional remedies take into account the interconnectedness of the mind, body, and spirit. This comprehensive approach recognizes that true healing involves addressing the root cause of an ailment, rather than just alleviating its symptoms.

Furthermore, the cultural and spiritual significance attached to these ancient remedies cannot be overlooked. For many indigenous communities, these remedies are not just about physical healing but also about preserving their cultural heritage and maintaining a sense of identity*. The rituals and practices associated with these remedies serve as a way to connect with their ancestors and honor their traditions.

In addition to their cultural and holistic aspects, ancient tribal remedies have also gained recognition in the scientific community. Researchers have started to explore the medicinal properties of various traditional herbs and plants, validating their effectiveness in treating certain conditions *. This growing body of scientific evidence further reinforces the continued significance of these remedies in modern times.

The relevance of ancient traditions in modern times is a fascinating subject to explore. The continued significance of ancient tribal remedies serves as a testament to their enduring value.

However, it is important to approach the topic of ancient tribal remedies with a balanced perspective. It is necessary to consult with healthcare professionals and use these remedies as complementary approaches to conventional treatments.

Holistic tribal remedies offer a unique perspective on healthcare that can complement modern practices. By exploring the integration of ancient traditions into contemporary healthcare systems, we can assess the potential benefits and challenges that arise.

One of the key benefits of incorporating holistic tribal remedies into modern healthcare is the emphasis on a holistic approach to wellness. As I've noted, tribal remedies often focus on treating the whole person, taking into account physical, mental, and spiritual aspects of health. This comprehensive approach can provide a more well-rounded and personalized healthcare experience for patients.

Additionally, tribal remedies often rely on natural and plant-based remedies, which can offer alternative treatment options for certain conditions, without many of the side effects of modern medicine*. Traditional healing practices, such as herbal medicine and acupuncture, have been used for centuries and may provide effective solutions for various ailments. Integrating these remedies into modern healthcare can expand the range of treatment options available to patients.

However, there are also challenges associated with integrating ancient traditions into contemporary healthcare systems. One challenge is the need for scientific validation and evidence-based research. While tribal remedies have been passed down through generations, meaning they clearly work for those communities, they may lack the rigorous scientific studies that modern medicine demands. Some may find it important to conduct research to validate the safety and efficacy of these remedies before integrating them into mainstream healthcare.

Another challenge is the potential clash of cultural beliefs and practices. Modern healthcare systems are often rooted in Western medicine, which may have different perspectives and approaches compared to tribal traditions. It is crucial to approach the integration of these traditions with cultural sensitivity and respect, ensuring that patients' beliefs and values are honored. This is something I believe has been lacking with the dominance of modern medicine.

The integration of holistic tribal remedies into modern healthcare requires collaboration and communication between different healthcare providers. This includes fostering partnerships between traditional healers and medical professionals to ensure a cohesive and coordinated approach to patient care. Building trust and understanding between these different healthcare systems is essential for successful integration.

Exploring how holistic tribal remedies can complement modern healthcare practices is an important endeavor, one that probably won't happen overnight. As our communities work on creating a more inclusive and comprehensive approach to health and well-being, we can take steps as women that put the power of our personal lives back into our own hands. In the next chapter we will look in depth at African American herbalism, with specific herbs you can explore incorporating.

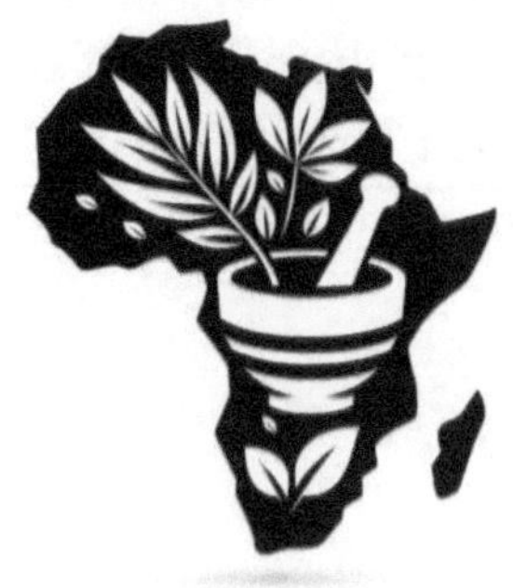

Chapter 2
African American Herbalism

In this chapter, we will uncover the rich heritage of African American herbalism. We will explore the traditional herbs and plants that have played a vital role in African American healing practices for generations. Many of these herbs are regaining recognition in the African American community today for their effectiveness.

Nature's bounty holds the key to wellness and vitality. We will learn about the unique methods and techniques employed by African American healers that harness the power of plants to restore balance and promote well-being.

This chapter is not just about the medicinal properties of herbs—it is a celebration of African American culture and its profound connection to herbal remedies. We will delve into the stories and traditions that have shaped the practice of herbalism within this vibrant community, recognizing the resilience and wisdom that have been preserved through the ages.

Let's begin this exploration, where the past intertwines with the present, and the healing power of nature is revealed in all its glory.

Plants of African American Herbal Medicine

Specific herbs and plants hold immense cultural significance in African American healing practices*. These natural remedies have been passed down through generations, carrying both medicinal properties and historical importance within the community. They serve as a connection to ancestral knowledge and traditions, representing resilience, spirituality, and the power of nature.

These healing practices not only address physical ailments but also promote holistic well-being. The utilization of these herbs and plants not only provides relief but also fosters a sense of cultural identity and pride, preserving and celebrating African American heritage.

Health, Herbs, Teas, and Hormone Balance

One such healing herb is Sassafras, known for its aromatic qualities and healing properties. It has been used for centuries in African American healing traditions to treat various ailments, including skin conditions and digestive issues*. Its distinct flavor and scent make it a popular ingredient in teas and tonics*.

One creative way to incorporate Sassafras into your recipes is by infusing it into a homemade syrup, adding a unique twist to your cocktails or drizzling it over pancakes and waffles made with healthy ingredients for a delightful breakfast treat.

Another notable plant is Echinacea, which has been valued for its immune-boosting properties*. African American healers have long recognized its ability to enhance the body's natural defenses and promote overall well-being. Echinacea is often incorporated into remedies to combat colds, flu, and other respiratory ailments.

Ginger, with its potent anti-inflammatory and digestive benefits, holds a prominent place in African American healing practices. It is revered for its ability to soothe upset stomachs, alleviate nausea, and reduce inflammation in the body*. Ginger tea is a common remedy used to promote digestion and relieve discomfort.

I personally love ginger, I take it on flights, when I'm having an upset stomach, or when I feel symptoms of a cold or sore throat arising. Almost every southern African household today still always has this plant, and many other herbs.

Mullein, a plant with soft, fuzzy leaves and vibrant yellow flowers, has been utilized in African American healing for its respiratory benefits*. It is often brewed into tea or used in steam inhalations to ease coughs, congestion, and respiratory discomfort.

Aloe vera is a succulent plant that has gained popularity for its numerous health benefits*. It is commonly used in skincare products due to its soothing and moisturizing properties. Aloe vera gel can help heal sunburns, cuts, and minor skin irritations*. When consumed internally, aloe vera juice may aid digestion, promote detoxification, and support a healthy immune system*. It is also believed to have anti-inflammatory effects and may help reduce symptoms of inflammatory conditions like arthritis. Forever Living is a brand that uses aloe vera as its primary ingredient for various healing drinks, it has become incredibly popular in African communities over the years.

Also known as Sambucus, Elderberry is a powerful plant that has been used for centuries in traditional medicine*. It is rich in antioxidants and vitamins, particularly vitamin C, which helps strengthen the immune system. Elderberry has been shown to have antiviral properties and may help reduce the duration and severity of cold and flu symptoms. Additionally, it has anti-inflammatory effects and may provide relief from allergies and respiratory conditions.

Yarrow, scientifically known as Achillea millefolium, is a versatile herb with a long history of medicinal use. It is known for its ability to support the body's natural healing processes*. Yarrow has anti-inflammatory and antimicrobial properties, making it useful for treating wounds, cuts, and bruises. It can also help alleviate digestive issues, such as bloating and indigestion. Furthermore, yarrow has been used to reduce fever and relieve menstrual cramps*.

African American Women have long been connected to nature and the art of healing and prolonged well-being. Many hormone balance assistance teas for women are formulated with a variety of these plants and herbs that are known to have beneficial effects on hormonal health*. These teas often contain a combination of carefully selected ingredients that work synergistically to support women. Other commonly used plants and herbs from around the world in these teas include:

1. Chasteberry (Vitex agnus-castus): Chasteberry is a popular herb that has been traditionally used to support female reproductive health*. It is believed to help regulate menstrual cycles and alleviate symptoms of premenstrual syndrome (PMS).

3. Black Cohosh (Actaea racemosa): Black Cohosh is a herb that has been used for centuries to support women's health, particularly during menopause. It is believed to help alleviate hot flashes, mood swings, and other menopausal symptoms.

4. Red Raspberry Leaf (Rubus idaeus): Red Raspberry Leaf is a popular herb that is believed to have toning and strengthening effects on the uterus and may help regulate menstrual cycles.

5. Maca Root (Lepidium meyenii): Maca root is a plant native to the Andes Mountains of Peru. It is known for its adaptogenic properties and is believed to help balance hormones, boost energy levels, and support overall well-being.

6. Licorice Root (Glycyrrhiza glabra): Licorice root is a herb that is often included in hormone balance teas for its potential benefits on hormonal health*. It is believed to have estrogen-like effects and may help alleviate symptoms of hormonal imbalances*.

By incorporating these plants and herbs into our daily lives, we can enhance our overall well-being and promote a proactive approach to health. However, it is important to consult with a healthcare professional before using any herbal remedies if you have any underlying medical conditions or are taking medications.

An Alternative Health Revolution

Taking another example, Kombucha is a fermented tea beverage that is gaining popularity in African and African American communities*.

Though I personally do find the hype extreme, this popularity can be attributed to its claimed associated health benefits and unique flavor profile.

Kombucha is made by fermenting sweetened tea with a symbiotic culture of bacteria and yeast (SCOBY)*. During the fermentation process, the SCOBY consumes the sugar in the tea and produces probiotics, enzymes, and organic acids, which contribute to its gut-health-promoting properties. The resulting beverage is fizzy, tangy, and often infused with various fruits or herbs for added flavor. Its growing popularity can also be attributed to its refreshing taste and its appeal as a trendy and alternative beverage option.

A number of people are waking up to the necessity for an alternative health revolution, though this often does result in a messy process of trying to enact this revolution. One example is the obsession of the African plant Zumbani that came with the onset of the coronavirus pandemic*. It is so essential to actually sit down and deeply explore both alternative and traditional medicine, and slowly begin putting it into practice in a reasonable and balanced way as communities.

A lot of these plants and herbs work primarily by boosting our immune systems and reinvigorating the life force energy that flows through our bodies. This innate holistic approach makes well-being primarily a preventative rather than cure-based approach.

The historical significance of these herbs and plants in African American culture cannot be overstated. They represent a connection to ancestral wisdom and a testament to the resilience and resourcefulness of African American healers throughout history.

By preserving and passing down these traditional healing practices, we continue to honor its heritage and empower healthier future generations. Now more than ever, with big pharma dominating the world, a return to holistic health is needed if we are to preserve the well-being and life-quality of humanity.

Unique Methods, Techniques, and Practices of African American Herbal Medicine

This section will delve into the unique methods and techniques employed in African American herbal medicine, shedding light on the preparation and administration of various herbal remedies.

One of the key aspects of African American herbal medicine is the use of different methods to extract the healing properties of plants. Infusions, for example, involve steeping herbs in hot water to create a potent herbal tea*. This method allows for the extraction of the plant's medicinal compounds, which can then be ingested for their therapeutic benefits. Infusions are often used to address common ailments such as colds, digestive issues, and stress.

Poultices are another important technique in African American herbal medicine. A poultice is a soft, moist mass made from crushed or ground herbs that is applied directly to the skin*. This method allows for the direct absorption of the plant's healing properties through the skin, providing relief for various conditions such as inflammation, wounds, and skin irritations. Poultices are typically made by combining herbs with a binding agent, such as clay or honey, to create a paste-like consistency that can be easily applied to the affected area*.

In addition to infusions and poultices, tinctures are widely used. A tincture is a concentrated liquid extract made by soaking herbs in alcohol or vinegar*. This method allows for the preservation of the plant's medicinal properties over a longer period of time. Tinctures are often taken orally by adding a few drops to water or other beverages. They are known for their effectiveness in addressing various health issues, including digestive disorders, respiratory ailments, and immune system support.

It is important to note that African American herbal medicine is not just about the methods and techniques used, but also about the cultural significance and spiritual connection to the plants. The process of extracting and utilizing the healing power of plants itself can be a sacred ritual that nourishes the mind and spirit. The holistic approach to planet medicine emphasizes the importance of understanding the plants' energetic properties and their relationship to the person seeking healing.

On this note, you can create your own healing ritual practices that can become regular moments of self-care. This is something we need today as our lives as women are often demanding and hectic, with little time and energy left dedicated to ourselves. We will come back to this in a moment, first let's take a look at traditional African American healing rituals and practices.

Traditional Healing Rituals and Practices

Traditional healing rituals and practices play a significant role in the holistic African herbal healing for women. These ancient customs, such as smudging and spiritual cleansing, still carry with them the wisdom and power of our ancestors. In this section, we will explore the profound impact of these rituals on the mind, body, and spirit of women seeking balance and well-being.

Smudging, a practice commonly found in many indigenous cultures, involves the burning of sacred herbs, such as sage or sweetgrass, to purify and cleanse the energy of a space or an individual. The fragrant smoke is believed to carry away negative energies, allowing positive vibrations to flow freely. For women, smudging can be a powerful tool for releasing emotional burdens, promoting clarity, and restoring inner harmony.

Spiritual cleansing is another integral aspect of traditional healing. It involves various rituals and ceremonies aimed at removing spiritual blockages and restoring spiritual balance. These practices often incorporate the use of herbs, crystals, and sacred objects to facilitate the release of stagnant energy and promote healing on a deep level. Women seeking holistic healing can benefit greatly from these rituals, as they provide a sacred space for introspection, self-discovery, and transformation. You can use spiritual cleansing for a person, space, or object.

There are numerous other traditional healing practices that are specifically tailored to address the unique needs of women. For example, herbal baths infused with medicinal plants and flowers can be used to promote physical and emotional well-being. These baths not only cleanse the body but also nourish the spirit, allowing you to reconnect with your innate wisdom and Divine Feminine power.

Furthermore, traditional healing rituals often incorporate the power of sound and music. Chanting, drumming, and singing can be used to create a sacred atmosphere and invoke the healing energies of the ancestors. These rhythmic vibrations have a profound effect on the body and mind, helping to release tension, reduce stress, and restore balance.

By embracing these ancient traditions, women can tap into their inner strength, cultivate self-care, and embark on a transformative journey towards holistic well-being. These time-honored customs provide a sacred space for women to reconnect with their roots, heal their bodies and spirits, and embrace their innate power.

You can integrate any and all of these practices into your own rituals as you embark on a transformative journey towards holistic well-being and reclaim your rightful place as a healer and catalyst in your community.

Personalized Lunar Eclipse Holistic Cleansing Ritual for Women

As women, we have a unique connection to the lunar cycle, as our own menstrual cycles often align with the phases of the moon (Lee, 2015). Harnessing the energy of a lunar eclipse can be a powerful opportunity for spiritual cleansing, holistic health, and emotional release (McCormick, 2020). This personalized ritual is designed to help you connect with the natural elements, engage in self-care, and embrace the transformative energy of the lunar eclipse.

Step 1: Setting the Intention. Find a quiet and comfortable space where you can perform the ritual undisturbed. Light a candle and take a few deep breaths to center yourself. Set your intention for the ritual, focusing on what you wish to release, heal, or manifest during this lunar eclipse.

Step 2: Herbal Bath. Prepare a warm herbal bath infused with cleansing and soothing herbs. Choose herbs such as lavender, chamomile, rosemary, or sage. Add a handful of these herbs to a muslin bag or directly to the bathwater. As you soak in the bath, visualize the water washing away any negative energy or emotional burdens you may be carrying.

Step 3: Balancing Teas. After your bath, prepare a cup of balancing tea to further support your holistic health. Choose herbal teas that promote relaxation, balance, and emotional well-being. Some options include chamomile, peppermint, lemon balm, or passionflower. Sip your tea mindfully, allowing its warmth and healing properties to nourish your body and spirit.

Step 4: Connecting with the Natural Elements. Step outside or open a window to connect with the natural elements during the lunar eclipse. Feel the earth beneath your feet, breathe in the fresh air, and observe the moon's transformation. Take a moment to reflect on the interconnectedness of all things and your own place within the universe.

Step 5: Sound Healing. Engage in sound healing to further enhance your spiritual cleansing. You can use singing bowls, chimes, or even your own voice. Close your eyes and focus on the vibrations and tones, allowing them to resonate within you. Visualize the sound waves clearing any stagnant energy and bringing harmony to your mind, body, and spirit.

Step 6: Emotional Release. Take a journal or a piece of paper and write down any emotions, thoughts, or experiences that you are ready to release. Allow yourself to express freely without judgment. Once you have written everything down, tear the paper into small pieces as a symbolic act of letting go. Dispose of the paper in a way that feels meaningful to you, such as burying it in the earth or burning it safely.

Step 7: Closing and Gratitude. As you conclude the ritual, express gratitude for the opportunity to connect with the lunar eclipse energy and engage in self-care. Blow out the candle, acknowledging the completion of the ritual. Take a moment to reflect on the insights gained and the intentions set during this sacred time.

Remember, this ritual is a personal and intuitive practice. Feel free to modify or adapt it to suit your own needs and preferences. May this lunar eclipse spiritual cleansing holistic health ritual bring you clarity, healing, and empowerment.

When looking at the cultural and historical context of African American herbal remedies, we become intimate with the rich and enduring legacy of these practices.

Throughout generations, African Americans have demonstrated a remarkable ability to preserve and pass down their herbal knowledge, ensuring its continuity and relevance in contemporary times. The significance of herbal remedies in African American cultural traditions cannot be overstated, as they not only serve as remedies for physical ailments but also as a means of promoting holistic well-being. These remedies are deeply rooted in the African diaspora, reflecting the resilience, resourcefulness, and wisdom of African American communities.

By embracing and continuing to explore the healing properties of herbs, African Americans are reclaiming our ancestral practices and reaffirming our cultural identity. Moreover, the utilization of herbal remedies fosters a sense of empowerment and self-sufficiency within these communities, as we are able to address their health needs in a natural and sustainable manner.

As we move forward, it is crucial to recognize and appreciate the contributions of African American herbal remedies to the broader field of holistic medicine. By acknowledging and integrating these practices into mainstream healthcare, we can create a more inclusive and comprehensive approach to well-being that honors the diverse cultural traditions that have shaped our society.

Through continued research, education, and advocacy, we can ensure that African American herbal remedies are not only preserved but also celebrated for their invaluable contributions to the health and wellness of individuals and communities alike.

In the next chapter, we will dive deeper into Black medicine for women's health.

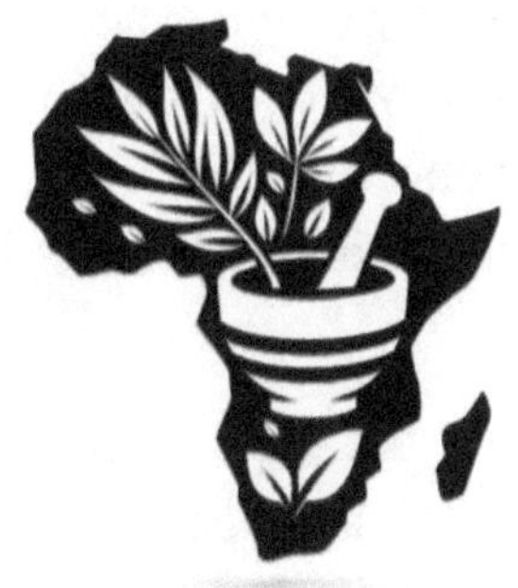

Chapter 3
Black Medicine for Women's Health

Black medicine has long been a powerful and transformative approach to women's holistic health. Have you ever explored the power of black medicine in nurturing women's vitality and internal harmony?

In this chapter, we will explore the realm of black medicine and its impact on women's well-being. We will uncover ancient remedies that promote women's health, from traditional practices to modern applications. Additionally, we will discuss specific black medicine remedies that have been beneficial for women throughout history. Furthermore, I'll highlight the important role of black medicine in addressing common women's health issues, providing insights and guidance for a holistic self-care routine.

Traditional black medicine remedies for women's health,beauty,and life force have been used for centuries to address various health concerns and promote overall well-being. Let's look at some of these practices in detail, including their benefits and effectiveness, as well as safety precautions.

Herbal Tinctures: As I briefly noted earlier, herbal tinctures are concentrated extracts made by soaking herbs in alcohol or a mixture of alcohol and water. They have been traditionally used by women to address common health concerns such as menopause symptoms, PMS, and hormonal imbalances. Some specific herbal tinctures used by women include:

Black Cohosh: Known for its potential to alleviate menopause symptoms like hot flashes, night sweats, and mood swings (The Health Benefits of Black Cohosh, 2019) (Huizen, 2017).

Chaste Tree Berry: Often used to regulate menstrual cycles, reduce PMS symptoms, and support hormonal balance (What Is Chasteberry, and What Can It Do?, 2022).

Dong Quai: Traditionally used to relieve menstrual cramps, regulate periods, and support reproductive health (Mayszak, 2018).

These herbal tinctures contain active compounds that may provide relief for women's health concerns. While scientific studies on their effectiveness are limited, anecdotal evidence and traditional use highlight their potential benefits.

To incorporate herbal tinctures into daily routines, women can follow the recommended dosage instructions provided by reputable herbalists or consult with a holistic healthcare professional.

Natural Skincare Remedies

Black medicine remedies for skin care focus on maintaining healthy and radiant skin. Women have used various natural remedies for centuries, including:

- Herbal Face Masks: Using herbs like turmeric, rose petals, or neem, women create masks to cleanse, nourish, and rejuvenate the skin.

- Infused Oils: Infusing natural oils with herbs like lavender, chamomile, or calendula can provide moisturizing and soothing effects for the skin.

- Natural Exfoliants: Ingredients like oatmeal, sugar, or coffee grounds are used to gently exfoliate the skin, removing dead cells and promoting a healthy glow.

These natural skincare remedies offer potential benefits such as improved skin texture, hydration, and reduced inflammation (Baghadia, 2023) (Goins, 2022). The use of herbal ingredients in skincare has been valued for their antioxidant, anti-inflammatory, and antimicrobial properties (Radhakrishnan, n.d.). Women can incorporate these remedies into their skincare routine by using them as masks, applying infused oils, or using natural exfoliants in a gentle manner.

Nourishing Tonics

Nourishing tonics made from holistic medicine ingredients are believed to support women's overall health and vitality (Snyder, 2021). These tonics often include adaptogenic herbs, roots, and a variety of mushrooms known for their potential to balance the body and promote well-being. You can often get them in holistic health stores, and you may also be supporting a Black Woman's small business.

Some examples include:

Ashwagandha: An adaptogenic herb that may help reduce stress, balance cortisol, and boost energy levels (Benefits of Ashwagandha and How Much to Take, 2022).

Reishi Mushroom: Known for its potential immune-boosting properties and ability to support overall well-being (Kubala, 2021).

Maca Root: Traditionally used to enhance energy, balance hormones, and support reproductive health (How to Use Maca for Hormone Balance, 2021).

These nourishing tonics can be consumed as teas, decoctions, or in powdered form. Women can incorporate these tonics into their daily routine by following recommended dosage instructions and consulting with a healthcare professional if necessary.

Ceremonial Practices

Black medicine remedies for women's health often encompass cultural and spiritual practices that have been passed down through generations. These rituals and practices hold significance beyond their physical effects and may include ceremonies, prayers, or specific traditions. They provide a holistic approach to women's health, addressing emotional, mental, and spiritual well-being.

The benefits of these rituals and practices promote a sense of connection, empowerment, and self-care. They can help women cultivate mindfulness, reduce stress, and enhance overall well-being. Incorporating these practices into daily routines can involve setting aside dedicated time for self-reflection, meditation, or engaging in activities that promote inner peace and balance.

Safety and Precautions

While traditional black medicine remedies for women's health have been used for generations, it's important to consider the following safety precautions:

- Consult with a Healthcare Professional: Before incorporating any new remedies into their routine, especially for pregnant or breastfeeding women or those with underlying health conditions, it's crucial to consult with a healthcare professional. They can provide personalized guidance and ensure compatibility with existing medications or treatments.

- Potential Side Effects: Some herbal remedies may have potential side effects or interactions with medications. It's important to be aware of any potential side effects and discontinue use if adverse reactions occur.

- Quality and Source: When using herbal tinctures or other remedies, ensure they are sourced from reputable suppliers and follow recommended dosage instructions. Quality and purity of ingredients are essential for safety and effectiveness.

All these remedies bring together communities, serving as a source of empowerment and self-care. They embody the wisdom and resilience of Black women.

Preserving and honoring traditional knowledge and practices related to black medicine remedies is crucial for future generations of women. By doing so, we ensure the continuity of cultural heritage and empower women to take control of their health and well-being. These remedies offer an alternative approach to self-care that is rooted in community, nature, and spirituality.

Furthermore, preserving traditional knowledge helps challenge the erasure and marginalization of Black women's contributions to healthcare. It acknowledges the expertise and wisdom that has been historically undervalued and overlooked. By honoring and sharing these practices, we uplift the voices and experiences of Black women, promoting inclusivity and equity in healthcare.

Understanding the Role of Black Medicine in Addressing Common Women's Health Issues

Black medicine, also known as traditional African medicine, has a rich history of addressing various health concerns (Kazmierczak, 2020). In recent years, there has been a growing interest in exploring the role of black medicine in addressing common women's health issues. It is important for me to shed light on how black medicine remedies can provide natural alternatives to conventional treatments and support overall women's health. I took a number of specific areas relating to women's health in all my books. Here are a few.

Menstrual Problems

Black medicine offers a holistic approach to managing menstrual problems. Traditional remedies, such as herbal teas and tinctures, have been used for centuries to alleviate menstrual pain, regulate irregular cycles, and reduce heavy bleeding. For example, herbs like dong quai and chaste tree berry are known for their ability to balance hormones and promote a healthy menstrual flow. Black medicine practitioners also emphasize the importance of lifestyle modifications, including stress reduction techniques and dietary changes, to support menstrual health.

From a holistic health and traditional African and Eastern perspective, women's menstrual cycles and energy levels are deeply interconnected. The menstrual cycle is not just a physical process but also a reflection of the energetic and emotional state of a woman (Walters, 2021). It is believed that the menstrual cycle is influenced by the ebb and flow of cosmic energies, as well as the internal balance of the body and mind.

In holistic health, the menstrual cycle is seen as a natural rhythm that mirrors the cycles of nature. Just as the moon waxes and wanes, so does a woman's energy throughout her cycle. During the menstrual phase, which is the bleeding phase, a woman's energy is typically lower as her body sheds the uterine lining (Walters, 2021). This is a time for rest, introspection, and self-care. It is important for women to honor their bodies' need for rest during this phase and listen to their intuition.

Women may experience the bleeding phase differently in terms of their energy levels and actions. One factor that can influence this is the timing of their menstrual cycle in relation to the lunar phases. For instance, some women may find that when they start their period during the full moon, they feel more energized and active, wanting to share their gifts with the world, they may also be more sexually activated (Walters, 2021). On the other hand, women who begin their cycle during the new moon phase might experience lower energy levels and may be more inclined to rest and conserve their energy, finding themselves in a reflective mood. A woman's typical cycle often changes over the course of her life.

As the menstrual cycle progresses into the follicular phase, which follows the menstrual phase, a woman's energy begins to rise. This is a time of new beginnings, creativity, and growth. Women may feel more energized, focused, and inspired during this phase. It is a great time for setting intentions, starting new projects, and engaging in physical activities. Typically, this phase aligns with the waxing crescent moon, which builds up following the new moon.

The ovulatory phase, which occurs around mid-cycle, is considered the peak of a woman's energy. This is when the body prepares for potential conception, and there is a surge of vitality and magnetism. Women may feel more outgoing, confident, and sexually charged during this phase. It is a time for socializing, connecting with others, and embracing one's sensuality.

Finally, the luteal phase, which follows ovulation, is a time of winding down and preparation for the next menstrual cycle. Energy levels may start to decline, and women may experience heightened emotions and introspection. It is important to honor the need for self-care, relaxation, and emotional support during this phase.

From an esoteric perspective, the menstrual cycle is seen as a sacred time of connection to the divine feminine energy. Many believe that during menstruation, women are more attuned to their intuition, spiritual insights, and emotional healing. It is a time for self-reflection, inner work, and connecting with the deeper aspects of oneself.

Hormonal Imbalances

Hormonal imbalances can cause a range of symptoms, including mood swings, acne, and irregular periods. African holistic health recognizes the interconnectedness of the body and aims to restore hormonal balance through natural means (African Holistic Health: A Comprehensive Guide, 2023).

Herbal remedies like maca root and black cohosh have been traditionally used to regulate hormones and alleviate symptoms associated with imbalances. Additionally, lifestyle recommendations, such as regular exercise and adequate sleep, are often incorporated to support hormonal health.

Fertility Challenges

Black medicine offers a unique perspective on fertility challenges, focusing on the overall well-being of the individual. Traditional practices often involve the use of specific herbs, such as red raspberry leaf and nettle, to support reproductive health (Baker, 2019). These herbs are believed to nourish the reproductive organs, balance hormones, and improve fertility. Black medicine practitioners also emphasize the importance of emotional and spiritual well-being, as stress and trauma can impact fertility. Techniques like meditation, counseling, and energy healing may be incorporated to address these aspects.

Menopausal Symptoms

The transition into menopause can bring about various physical and emotional changes. Black medicine recognizes this natural phase of a woman's life and offers remedies to alleviate menopausal symptoms. Herbs like black cohosh and evening primrose oil are commonly used to reduce hot flashes, mood swings, and intimate care/.

Additionally, lifestyle modifications, including a nutrient-rich diet and regular exercise, are encouraged to support overall well-being during this transition.

I explore how women can holistically thrive through menopause in-depth in my book The Black Woman's Guide to Menopause which is specifically dedicated to this topic.

Incorporating Black Medicine into a Holistic Self-Care Routine

When it comes to holistic self-care, incorporating black medicine can be a powerful addition to your wellness routine. Black medicine refers to natural remedies derived from plants, herbs, and other sources that have been traditionally used for their healing properties. However, it is important to approach black medicine with caution and respect, as it can have potent effects on the body and interact with other medications or conditions.

One key aspect to consider when incorporating black medicine into your self-care routine is the method of preparation. Different plants and herbs may require specific preparation techniques such as brewing teas, creating tinctures, or making poultices. Researching and understanding the appropriate preparation methods for each black medicine remedy is crucial to ensure its effectiveness and safety.

Dosage is another important consideration. Black medicine remedies often have recommended dosages based on factors such as age, weight, and health conditions. It is essential to follow these guidelines to avoid potential side effects or adverse reactions. Consulting with a healthcare professional or traditional healer who is knowledgeable about black medicine can provide valuable guidance on appropriate dosages for your specific needs.

Furthermore, it is crucial to be aware of potential interactions or contraindications. Some black medicine remedies may interact negatively with certain medications or exacerbate existing health conditions. It is important to disclose all medications and health conditions to your healthcare professional or traditional healer to ensure safe integration of black medicine into your self-care routine.

Lastly, consulting with healthcare professionals and traditional healers is highly recommended when incorporating black medicine remedies into your self-care practice. They can provide personalized guidance, monitor your progress, and address any concerns or questions you may have. Their expertise and experience can help you navigate the complexities of black medicine and ensure its integration into your holistic self-care routine is safe and effective.

Incorporating black medicine into your holistic self-care routine can be a transformative experience. By following proper preparation methods, appropriate dosages, and seeking guidance from healthcare professionals and traditional healers, you can harness the power of black medicine to enhance your well-being and promote a balanced and harmonious life.

In the next chapter we will pivot slightly as we focus on reviving our Divine Feminine Energy.

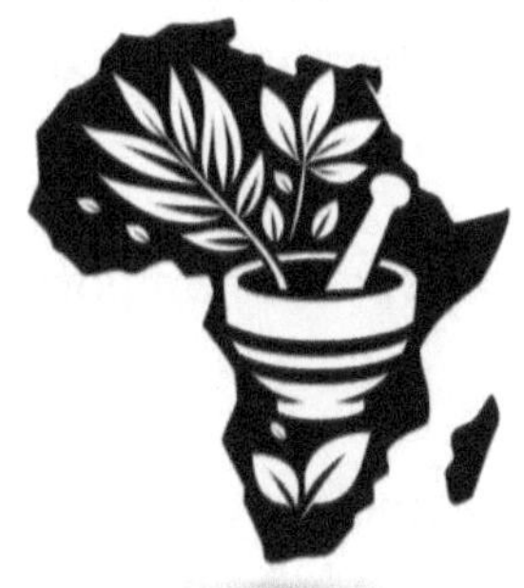

Chapter 4
Reviving Divine Feminine Energy

In a world where the hustle and bustle of everyday life often leaves us feeling disconnected and out of touch with our true selves, there is a profound need to explore the concept of divine feminine energy. This chapter invites you on a transformative journey, one that delves deep into the essence of the Divine Feminine and its vital role in our overall healing.

Within these pages, we will unravel the mysteries of the Divine Feminine shedding light on its significance and power. We will explore the practices and rituals that can awaken and nurture this sacred energy within each of us, allowing it to flow freely and harmoniously.

The Divine Feminine is not limited to gender. This is a universal force that resides within all beings. She represents qualities such as intuition, compassion, creativity, and nurturing. By embracing and honoring the Divine Feminine, we tap into a wellspring of wisdom and strength that can guide us towards a more balanced and fulfilling life.

Throughout this chapter, we will delve into ancient wisdom and modern insights, weaving together a tapestry of knowledge that will empower you to reclaim your divine feminine essence. We will explore the dance between Divine Masculine (DM) and Divine Feminine energies, seeking to find a harmonious equilibrium that brings forth wholeness and unity.

Understanding the Concept and Importance of Divine Feminine Energy

The concept of Divine Feminine energy holds profound significance in the realm of personal and collective healing. Embracing and harnessing this powerful energy can bring about transformative changes in our lives and society as a whole.

Divine feminine energy is a force that exists within both men and women, transcending gender boundaries (Patel, 2021). By acknowledging and honoring this energy, we can tap into immense potential for growth, healing, and empowerment.

One of the key reasons why embracing Divine Feminine energy is important is to restore balance. In a world that has long been dominated by masculine energy, characterized by competition, aggression, and control, the Divine Feminine offers a counterbalance of harmony, empathy, and collaboration. By integrating qualities of the DF into our lives, we can create a more harmonious and compassionate society.

Embracing the Divine Feminine allows us to reconnect with our inner wisdom. In a fast-paced and often chaotic world, we may find ourselves disconnected from our true selves and the guidance that lies within. By embracing the Divine Feminine, we can tap into our intuitive abilities, accessing a deeper understanding of ourselves and the world around us.

Embracing and Harnessing the Power of Divine Feminine Energy for Personal and Collective Healing

The significance of embracing and harnessing the power of Divine Feminine energy for personal and collective healing cannot be overstated. The Divine Feminine represents a powerful force that resides within each individual and has the potential to bring about profound transformation and healing on both personal and societal levels.

At its core, the Divine Feminine embodies characteristics that are often associated with the feminine aspect of our being, but they are not limited to any specific gender. Embracing and cultivating these qualities allows individuals to tap into a deeper sense of self-awareness, empathy, and connection with others.

One of the key aspects of the Divine Feminine is its nurturing nature. This nurturing energy is not only directed towards others but also towards oneself. By embracing the Divine Feminine, women learn to prioritize self-care and self-love, recognizing that their own well-being is essential for their ability to contribute positively to the world around them. This self-nurturing aspect of the Divine Feminine is crucial for personal healing and growth.

In addition to nurturing, the Divine Feminine is closely associated with compassion. Compassion is the ability to understand and empathize with the suffering of others, and it is a powerful tool for healing both individually and collectively. When we tap into Divine Feminine energy, we become more attuned to the needs and struggles of others, fostering a sense of unity and interconnectedness. This compassion allows for the healing of deep wounds and the building of supportive and nurturing communities.

Intuition is another significant aspect of the Divine Feminine. Intuition is the inner knowing that goes beyond logical reasoning and taps into a deeper wisdom. By embracing and harnessing the power of intuition, we can make decisions that are aligned with our authentic selves and our highest good. Intuition also serves as a guide for personal healing, helping women navigate our inner landscape and uncover hidden truths.

Creativity is yet another quality associated with the divine feminine. Creativity is not limited to artistic expression but encompasses the ability to think outside the box, find innovative solutions, and bring forth new ideas. By embracing our creative potential, women can tap into a limitless source of inspiration and self-expression.

On a collective level, embracing and harnessing the power of Divine Feminine energy can lead to societal transformation and healing. The qualities of nurturing, compassion, intuition, and creativity are essential for building a more harmonious and balanced world. By valuing and honoring the Divine Feminine within ourselves and others, we create space for healing, understanding, and collaboration.

By embodying the qualities associated with the Divine Feminine, individuals can tap into their inner wisdom, nurture themselves and others, and contribute to the creation of a more compassionate and harmonious world. It is through the integration of the divine feminine that we can experience profound transformation and healing on both individual and societal levels.

Examples of Divine Feminine Energy in Cultural and Spiritual Traditions

The concept of divine feminine energy transcends cultural and spiritual boundaries, manifesting in various forms across different traditions. It's important to look at examples from diverse cultural and spiritual backgrounds to illustrate the multifaceted interpretations of Divine Feminine energy. Through these examples, we can gain a deeper understanding of how this energy is revered and celebrated across the world.

1. Hinduism: In Hinduism, the Divine Feminine is personified as various goddesses, such as "Durga, Lakshmi, and Saraswati" (hridoyjitgogoi@gmail.com, 2023, p.2). Durga represents strength and protection, Lakshmi symbolizes abundance and prosperity, while Saraswati embodies wisdom and knowledge. These goddesses are worshiped and revered for their unique

qualities, reflecting different aspects of the divine feminine energy.

2. Ancient Egypt: In ancient Egyptian mythology, the goddess Isis is a prominent figure associated with Divine Feminine energy. She is revered as the mother goddess, representing fertility, magic, and healing (Lana, 2020). Isis is often depicted as a nurturing and protective figure, embodying the qualities of love, compassion, and wisdom.

3. Native American Traditions: Native American cultures have long recognized the presence of the Divine Feminine. For example, the Lakota people honor the White Buffalo Calf Woman, who is believed to have brought sacred teachings and spiritual guidance (Mark, 2023). She represents purity, harmony, and the interconnectedness of all living beings.

4. Buddhism: In Buddhism, the concept of the Divine Feminine is embodied in the figure of Tara, a bodhisattva associated with fierce compassion, strength, and enlightenment (Kane, 2021). Tara is revered as a powerful Divine Feminine deity, offering guidance and protection to those who seek her blessings. One of my favorite lines from her

5. Greek Mythology: Greek mythology portrays various goddesses who embody different aspects of the Divine Feminine. For instance, Aphrodite represents love and beauty, Athena symbolizes wisdom and strategy, and Artemis embodies independence and the wild aspects of nature. These goddesses reflect the diverse facets of feminine energy and serve as powerful archetypes in Greek mythology.

The important thing we discover along our journey is that Divine Feminine energy resides within us. The DF is not an external figure to be worshiped, though we can celebrate and honor her work.

While many patriarchal western religions that require us to worship an external figure and put this God above our lives, seeing him as pure and all powerful while we are weaker and in most cases "sinful", connecting with the Divine Feminine provides women with a new lens for their spiritual journey. They get to experience holistic empowerment, and the divinity and splendor that is within them. No longer are you waiting for an external savior, for you are in charge of your own life, health, and well-being. A true divine figure inspires you to see that you yourself are sacred, whole, and good enough.

It is crucial to recognize and embrace the inherent divine feminine energy that exists within each individual. By acknowledging that this Divine Feminine energy is an integral part of our being, we can tap into her power and potential for personal growth and empowerment.

Holistic empowerment of women involves nurturing and honoring the Divine Feminine energy within ourselves and others. It goes beyond external factors and societal expectations, focusing on the holistic well-being of women in all aspects of their lives - physical, emotional, mental, and spiritual. This empowerment encourages women to embrace their unique strengths, talents, and perspectives, and to express themselves authentically.

Through holistic empowerment, women can cultivate self-love, self-acceptance, and self-confidence.

This involves breaking free from limiting beliefs and societal norms that may hinder our progress. By recognizing and valuing our own worth, we can assert ourselves, set boundaries, and make choices that align with our true desires and aspirations. All the while uplifting and becoming closer to each other.

By doing so, we can create a world where women are valued, respected, and empowered to reach their full potential.

Exploring Practices and Rituals to Awaken and Nurture the Divine Feminine Within

There are specific practices and rituals that can assist women in connecting with and cultivating our Divine Feminine energy. By incorporating these techniques into our lives, we can awaken and nurture the Divine Feminine within us.

Meditation is a powerful tool for connecting with the divine feminine energy within. By setting aside dedicated time for meditation, we can create a sacred space to explore our inner selves and tap into our DF essence. During meditation, one can focus on visualizations that embody the qualities of the Divine Feminine, such as compassion, intuition, and creativity. This practice allows us to deepen our connection with these aspects of ourselves and invite presence into our daily lives.

Visualization exercises are another effective way to awaken and nurture the Divine Feminine within. Through visualization, individuals can create vivid mental images that align with the qualities they wish to embody. For example, one can visualize themselves surrounded by a soft, nurturing light, symbolizing the nurturing aspect of the Divine Feminine. By regularly engaging in visualization exercises, individuals can reinforce their connection with DF energy and integrate it into their being.

In addition to meditation and visualization, there are various other techniques that can support the awakening and nurturing of the inner goddess. Journaling, for instance, provides a space for self-reflection and exploration of one's emotions and experiences. By expressing thoughts and feelings on paper, we can gain a deeper understanding of ourselves and our sacred connection to the Divine Feminine. This practice can also serve as a tool for releasing any limiting beliefs or societal conditioning that may hinder the expression of DF energy.

Engaging in creative activities is another powerful way to awaken and nurture the DF within. Whether it's painting, dancing, writing, or any other form of artistic expression, these activities allow women to tap into their innate creativity and connect with their authentic selves.

By engaging in creative endeavors, we can channel the Divine Feminine and bring forth our unique gifts and talents into the world.

Self-care and self-love play a vital role in the process of embracing the Divine Feminine. Taking care of one's physical, emotional, and spiritual well-being is essential for nurturing this energy. This can involve practices such as nourishing the body with healthy food, engaging in regular exercise, practicing mindfulness, and setting boundaries to protect one's energy. By prioritizing self-care and self-love, we create a foundation of love and acceptance from which the Divine Feminine can flourish.

Exploring practices and rituals to awaken and nurture the Divine Feminine within is a transformative journey of self-discovery and empowerment. Through meditation, visualization exercises, journaling, creative activities, and self-care practices, women can deepen their connection with the divine feminine energy and embody its qualities in their daily lives.

It is so important to get back in touch with our DF essence, and learn how to balance this with DM qualities.

Learning How to Balance and Harmonize Masculine and Feminine Energies

The concept of balancing and harmonizing masculine and feminine energies is a topic of great significance in today's society. There exists a need for balance and harmony between these energies, not only within individuals but also in society as a whole. By exploring the challenges and misconceptions often associated with gender roles, as well as the importance of embracing and integrating both masculine and feminine qualities, we can gain a deeper understanding of this crucial aspect of personal and societal growth.

The philosophy of yin and yang embodies the concept of uniting the Divine Masculine and Feminine aspects within oneself, leading to a profound sense of wholeness, contentment, energetic harmony, and overall well-being. In some traditional Eastern and African communities it was believed that by embracing and balancing these opposing forces, we can achieve a state of inner equilibrium and spiritual growth. This idea emphasizes the importance of recognizing and integrating both the creative, intention driven will within us, and the action-oriented qualities within us, allowing us to tap into our full potential.*

By harmonizing these complementary energies, we unlock a deeper understanding of ourselves and cultivate a profound connection with the universe, ultimately leading to a more fulfilling and balanced life.

One of the primary challenges in achieving balance and harmony between masculine and feminine energies lies in the deeply ingrained societal expectations and stereotypes surrounding gender roles. Historically, society has assigned certain traits and behaviors as either masculine or feminine, creating a dichotomy that limits individuals' self-expression and potential. This rigid categorization often leads to a disconnection from one's authentic self and a suppression of certain qualities deemed incompatible with societal norms.

However, it is essential to recognize that masculine and feminine energies exist within all individuals, regardless of their biological sex or gender identity. Masculine energy is often associated with assertiveness, reason-based perception, and physical strength, while feminine energy embodies qualities such as intuition, emotion and sensory based perception, and empathy. This is the most simplified and basic expression of these energies, which are in fact much more complex, especially in the case of DF energy. Both energies are equally valuable and necessary for personal growth and the well-being of society.

By embracing and integrating both masculine and feminine qualities, women can tap into their full potential and experience a more balanced and fulfilling life. This integration allows for a greater range of self-expression, emotional intelligence, and adaptability. It enables us to navigate challenges with resilience and empathy, fostering healthier relationships and a more harmonious society.

Moreover, achieving balance and harmony between masculine and feminine energies is not limited to individuals alone. It is equally important for society as a whole to recognize and value the contributions of both energies. There is a difference between the energies of masculine and feminine, and imposed gender roles that are assigned by society according to one's sex. By breaking free from the confines of traditional gender roles, we can create a more inclusive and equitable society that celebrates diversity and fosters collaboration.

Learning how to balance and harmonize masculine and feminine energies is a transformative journey that requires self-reflection, openness, and a willingness to challenge societal norms. There are a number of ways we can begin putting this integration into practice. Let's take a look at a few.

Strategies and techniques for achieving balance and harmony between divine feminine and divine masculine energies within, to live a more empowered, holistic life as women can be transformative. By embracing both aspects of our being, we can tap into our full potential and experience a deeper sense of fulfillment. Here are some strategies and techniques to help you on this journey:

1. Self-reflection and awareness: Take time to reflect on your own beliefs, values, and behaviors related to femininity and masculinity. Explore how these aspects manifest in your life and identify any imbalances or biases. Developing self-awareness is the first step towards achieving balance. Journalling is one technique that assists with this reflection. You can try out the following journal prompts to help you explore your own beliefs, values, and behaviors related to femininity and masculinity:

1. How would you define femininity and masculinity? What characteristics or qualities do you associate with each?

2. Reflect on your upbringing and the messages you received about femininity and masculinity. How have these messages influenced your beliefs and behaviors?

3. What societal expectations or stereotypes do you feel pressure to conform to in terms of femininity and masculinity? How do these expectations impact your sense of self?

4. Consider the role models or influences in your life who embody femininity and masculinity. How have they shaped your understanding of these concepts?

5. Reflect on any personal experiences or moments that challenged your beliefs or assumptions about femininity and masculinity. How did these experiences impact your perspective?

6. How do your beliefs about femininity and masculinity align with your own values and principles? Are there any conflicts or contradictions?

7. Explore any biases or prejudices you may hold towards certain expressions of femininity or masculinity. How do these biases affect your interactions with others?

8. Consider the ways in which your beliefs about femininity and masculinity have evolved over time. What factors or experiences contributed to these changes?

9. Reflect on the impact of societal norms and expectations on your own self-expression and identity. How do you navigate these influences while staying true to yourself?

10. Imagine a world where femininity and masculinity were not defined by rigid stereotypes. How would this impact your own beliefs and behaviors?

1. Embrace your feminine energy: Cultivate practices that connect you with your uninhibited, sensual, emotionally aware, intuitive, and creative essence. This can include activities like reading or writing, dancing, painting, or spending time in nature. Allow yourself to express your emotions freely and honor your intuition.

2. Cultivate your masculine energy: Recognize the importance of your masculine energy and its positive qualities such as self-protection, reason-based actions, and physical strength. You can practice setting boundaries in your personal and professional life as you learn to say no, stand up for, and prioritize yourself. You can also engage in activities that promote material gain, public recognition, self-discipline, goal-setting, and problem-solving. This can involve physical exercise, learning new skills, taking on leadership roles, and taking charge of your financial

documentation and strategies. Balancing your masculine energy will empower you to take action and manifest your desires, leading to personal satisfaction, while simultaneously being connected to more relational, creative, and spirited actions of life, leading to interconnectedness and contentment. We are naturally healthier and happier when our lives are balanced and we feel capable of attaining and enjoying the lives we desire.

3. Seek support and guidance: Connect with like-minded individuals or seek guidance from mentors who have successfully integrated their divine feminine and masculine energies. Surrounding yourself with a supportive community can provide valuable insights and encouragement on your journey towards balance and harmony.

4. Practice mindfulness and meditation: Incorporate mindfulness and meditation into your daily routine. These practices can help you cultivate inner peace, clarity, and a deeper connection with your true self. By quieting the mind and focusing on the present moment, you can align your energies and create a harmonious inner state.

5. Embrace the power of rituals: Create rituals that honor both your divine feminine and masculine energies. This can include rituals for self-care, self-love, and self-expression. Engaging in rituals can help you establish a sense of sacredness and bring balance to your daily life.

6. Embody the qualities you seek: Strive to embody the qualities you wish to cultivate within yourself. Whether it's compassion, strength, or creativity, consciously practice these qualities in your interactions with others and in your daily life. By embodying these qualities, you will naturally attract more balance and harmony into your life.

Remember, achieving balance and harmony between divine feminine and divine masculine energies is a personal journey. It requires self-reflection, patience, and a commitment to personal growth. By embracing both aspects of your being, you can live a more empowered, holistic life as a woman.

African American women often embody this wholeness innately. Having both personal boundaries, strength, and ambition, all the while taking care of their communities and loved ones.

Not only is physical wellness and strength important, we also need to build the muscles of mental wellness, spiritual health, and emotional satisfaction. In the next chapter, we will look at Ancient Tribal Remedies for Emotional Wellness.

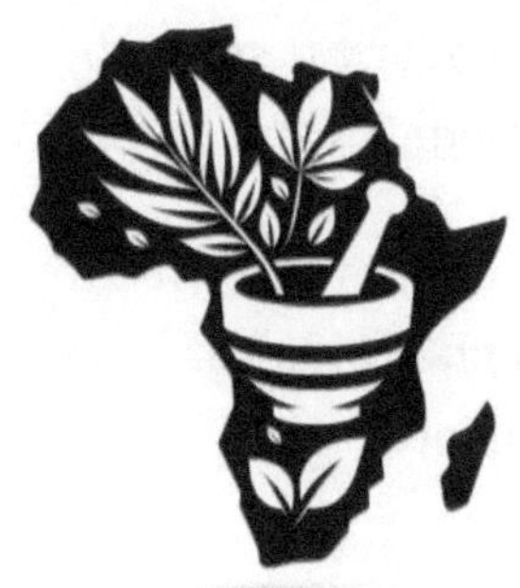

Chapter 5
Ancient Tribal Remedies for Emotional Wellness

Ancient tribal remedies for emotional healing and well-being is something that is only now being appreciated in the mainstream. Yet emotional health is so essential, it is the pillar of our life force energy.

In this chapter, we will discover remedies that have withstood the test of time, providing relief from psycho-emotional challenges such as stress, anxiety, and depression, to name a few. Through techniques to promote emotional balance and overall wellness, we will uncover the secrets of managing and overcoming these emotional burdens. Additionally, we will explore the connection between emotions and physical health, understanding how emotional, mental, spiritual, and physical wellness are interconnected.

Understanding the Connection Between Emotions and Physical Health

Emotions and physical health are deeply intertwined, forming a complex relationship that has been recognized by ancestral wisdom across cultures. This section delves into the intricate connection between emotions and physical well-being, highlighting the profound impact they have on each other.

Emotional well-being plays a significant role in maintaining good physical health. When we experience positive emotions such as joy, love, and contentment, our bodies respond by releasing hormones that promote overall well-being.. These hormones, including endorphins, oxytocin, and dopamine can boost our immune system, reduce inflammation, and enhance our ability to heal.

Conversely, negative emotions such as stress, anger, and sadness can have detrimental effects on our physical health. Prolonged stress, for instance, can lead to chronic inflammation, weakened immune function, and increased risk of various diseases. It can also disrupt sleep patterns, impair digestion, and contribute to the development of conditions like high blood pressure and heart disease.

The mind-body connection is a powerful force that should not be underestimated. Our thoughts and emotions can influence the functioning of our organs, nervous system, and immune response. For example, chronic stress can trigger the release of stress hormones like cortisol, which, when elevated over time, can disrupt the balance of our body's systems and contribute to the development of chronic illnesses.

Scientific evidence supports the mind-body connection through various studies and research. One study conducted by researchers at Harvard Medical School found that individuals who practiced mindfulness meditation experienced changes in brain activity and structure, indicating the impact of the mind on the physical body. Another study published in the Journal of Psychosomatic Medicine demonstrated that positive emotions, such as happiness and gratitude, were associated with improved cardiovascular health.

Furthermore, the link between the mind and our emotions is an intricate matter. Our emotions are a product of our thoughts and perceptions, and they can significantly influence our mental and physical well-being. When we experience positive emotions like joy or love, our bodies release neurotransmitters such as dopamine and serotonin, which promote feelings of happiness and relaxation. On the other hand, negative emotions like anger or sadness can activate the body's stress response, leading to physiological changes like increased heart rate and elevated blood pressure.

Understanding this link can empower individuals to prioritize their mental well-being and adopt practices that promote a harmonious balance between the mind and body.

Furthermore, physical health issues can also impact our emotional well-being. Dealing with chronic pain, illness, or disability can lead to feelings of frustration, sadness, and even depression. The burden of physical ailments can affect our self-esteem, relationships, and overall quality of life.

Recognizing the interplay between emotions and physical health is crucial for holistic well-being. By nurturing our emotional well-being, we can positively influence our physical health and vice versa. Engaging in activities that promote emotional balance, such as mindfulness, meditation, and therapy, can help reduce stress, improve mood, and enhance overall health.

The connection between emotions and physical health is undeniable. Nurturing this intricate relationship, we can strive for optimal well-being and lead healthier, more fulfilling lives.

Ancient tribal remedies have long been revered for their ability to restore balance and improve both emotional and physical health. These remedies offer unique insights into the holistic approach to well-being.

Unlike modern medicine, which often treats symptoms in isolation, tribal remedies recognize that emotional and physical health are deeply intertwined. By addressing the root causes of imbalance, they aim to restore harmony to the entire being.

Emotional health is a vital component of overall well-being, and ancient tribal remedies offer valuable insights into nurturing it. Practices such as meditation, herbal remedies, and ritualistic ceremonies help individuals connect with their inner selves and find inner peace. These remedies encourage self-reflection, emotional release, and the cultivation of positive emotions, leading to improved mental and emotional states.

Physical health is equally important, and ancient tribal remedies provide a wealth of knowledge in this area. Herbal remedies, for example, harness the healing properties of plants to address various ailments. From soothing digestive issues to boosting the immune system, as we have seen earlier, these remedies offer natural alternatives to synthetic medications. Additionally, practices like massage, acupuncture, and energy healing techniques help restore balance to the body's energy systems, promoting physical well-being.

The wisdom of ancient tribal remedies lies in their holistic approach to health.

Learning techniques to promote emotional balance and well-being

Ancient tribes have long recognized the importance of emotional balance and overall well-being. Through their wisdom and connection to nature, they developed various techniques and practices to promote emotional well-being. These time-honored methods can still be valuable in our modern lives. Here are some techniques employed by ancient tribes to promote emotional balance and well-being:

Meditation and Mindfulness: Ancient tribes understood the power of quieting the mind and being present in the moment. They practiced meditation and mindfulness to cultivate inner peace and emotional stability. By focusing on their breath or a specific object, they were able to calm their minds and find balance within. The power of taming the mind and sitting in stillness with full awareness cannot be overstated, it is a reprieve from the modern chaos of life.*that is acknowledge in *As a beginner to mindfulness and meditation, it helps to choose an anchor that you return your awareness to each time your mind wonders. This can be sound, bodily sensations, your breath, or a chosen crystal. It is natural for the mind to wonder, noticing when it does, and regularly bringing your attention back to your anchor, is where the shift happens.

It is like mental exercise that always allows you to tune in and be aware of your emotions and thoughts without judgment and attachment.

Connection with Nature: Ancient tribes recognized the healing power of nature. They spent time in natural surroundings, such as forests, mountains, or bodies of water, to restore their emotional well-being. They believed that being in harmony with the natural world helped them connect with their own inner selves. Connecting with nature can be joined with a mindfulness or meditation practice for even more emotional and mental healing.

Artistic Expression: Ancient African tribes embraced artistic expression as a means of emotional release and self-discovery. They engaged in activities such as painting, dancing, singing, and drumming to express their emotions and connect with their inner selves. These creative outlets allowed them to channel their energy and find emotional balance. A lot of these practices are still prevalent in holistic African communities today.

Rituals and Ceremonies: Rituals and ceremonies played a significant role in ancient tribal cultures. These practices provided a sense of belonging, purpose, and emotional grounding. Whether it was a sacred dance, a fire ceremony, or a communal gathering, these rituals allowed women to express their emotions, release negativity, and foster a sense of unity. A ritual is simply a regular or cyclical activity, with a specific intention, that brings you into deeper connection with yourself and the world around you.

Herbal Remedies: Because ancient tribes had such a deep understanding of the healing properties of plants and herbs., these were included in the realm of emotional healing as well. They used various herbal remedies to support emotional well-being the same way they did for physical wellness. For example, lavender was known for its calming effects, while chamomile helped reduce anxiety. These natural remedies were integrated into their daily lives to promote emotional balance.

Storytelling and Wisdom Sharing: Ancient tribes passed down their knowledge and wisdom through storytelling. They recognized the power of narratives in helping humans process their emotions and gain insights into their own experiences. By sharing stories of triumph, loss, and resilience, they provided guidance and inspiration for emotional well-being. Storytelling, when done correctly and in a guided form, can also help process relational trauma. Human beings are fortunate to be the only sentient beings with the capacity for deep emotional and mental processing, it comes naturally for us to make sense of things, tell stories, and use these capacities. Storytelling is a healing art.

Community Support: Ancient African tribes, particularly those with matriarchal values, valued the importance of community and social connections. They understood that a strong support system was essential for emotional balance. They relied on each other for emotional support, encouragement, and guidance during challenging times. This sense of belonging and interconnectedness contributed to their overall well-being. Community is still the centerpiece of most African and African American communities today, with the concept of "Ubuntu"(meaning "I am because we are") shared with all people in every area of life.

By exploring and incorporating these ancient techniques into our modern lives, we can cultivate emotional balance and overall well-being. The wisdom of ancient tribes serves as a reminder that emotional well-being is a holistic journey that requires nurturing our minds, bodies, and spirits.

Incorporating Techniques for Managing Emotions into Daily Life

Managing emotions is an essential skill that can greatly improve our overall well-being. By incorporating specific techniques such as breathing exercises and mindfulness practices into our daily lives, we can develop a greater sense of emotional balance and resilience. Consistency and regular practice are key to achieving optimal results.

Here is a step-by-step guide on how to incorporate these techniques into your daily routine:

- Set aside dedicated time: Begin by allocating a specific time each day for practicing these techniques. It could be in the morning, during a lunch break, or before bedtime. Consistency is crucial, so choose a time that works best for you and commit to it.

- Start with breathing exercises each morning: Find a quiet and comfortable space where you can sit or lie down. Close your eyes and take a deep breath in through your nose, allowing your abdomen to expand. Hold the breath for a few seconds, and then exhale slowly through your mouth. Repeat this process for a few minutes, focusing solely on your breath. This simple exercise helps calm the mind and relax the body.

- Integrate mindfulness into daily activities: Mindfulness involves being fully present in the moment and non-judgmentally observing your thoughts and emotions. Practice mindfulness during routine activities such as eating, walking, or even washing dishes. Pay attention to the sensations, smells, and tastes, and let go of any distractions. This cultivates a sense of awareness and helps manage emotions more effectively.

- Create reminders: To ensure consistency, set reminders or cues throughout the day to prompt you to practice these techniques. It could be a gentle alarm on your phone, sticky notes placed strategically, or associating the practice with specific activities like brushing your teeth or taking a break.

- Seek support: Consider joining a meditation or mindfulness group, or find an accountability partner who shares your interest in managing emotions. Connecting with others who are on a similar journey can provide encouragement and motivation.

- Be patient and kind to yourself: Remember that managing emotions is a lifelong practice. It takes time and effort to develop new habits. If you miss a day or find it challenging, don't be too hard on yourself. Embrace the process and celebrate small victories along the way.

By incorporating breathing exercises and mindfulness practices into your daily routine, you can gradually develop emotional resilience and enhance your overall well-being. Consistency and regular practice are the keys to unlocking the full potential of these techniques. So, start today and embark on a journey towards emotional balance and self-discovery.

Exploring Remedies for Managing Stress, Anxiety, and Depression

In today's fast-paced and demanding world, stress, anxiety, and depression have become prevalent issues affecting many Women. While modern medicine offers effective treatments, exploring traditional tribal remedies can provide valuable insights into alternative approaches for managing these emotional challenges.

There are various traditional tribal remedies used for alleviating stress, anxiety, and low moods. Specific herbs, plants, and rituals that have been traditionally employed. As always, although beneficial and effective, precautions and considerations need to be taken when using these remedies. It is best to use these as a preventative approach—a way of life. When using them as a potential remedy for any existing emotional or mental difficulty, always use them complementarity to traditional health care and modern therapy.

Emotional Self-care Herbal Remedies

Traditional tribal communities have long relied on the healing properties of herbs to address emotional imbalances. Here are a couple of examples:

- St. John's Wort (Hypericum perforatum): This herb has been used for centuries to alleviate symptoms of depression and anxiety. Its active compounds, such as hypericin and hyperforin, are believed to enhance serotonin levels in the brain, promoting a sense of well-being. However, it is important to note that St. John's Wort may interact with certain medications, so consulting a healthcare professional is advised.

- Ashwagandha (Withania somnifera): Ashwagandha, an adaptogenic herb, is known for its stress-reducing properties. It helps regulate cortisol levels, the hormone associated with stress, and promotes a calm and balanced state of mind. While generally safe, pregnant or breastfeeding individuals should consult a healthcare provider before using ashwagandha.

Plant-based Emotional Self-care Remedies

Traditional tribal communities have also utilized various plants to address emotional well-being. Here are a few examples:

- Lavender (Lavandula angustifolia): Lavender is renowned for its calming and soothing effects. Its aromatic properties have been shown to reduce anxiety and promote relaxation. Whether used in essential oil form, as a tea, or in bath products, lavender can be a valuable tool in managing stress and anxiety.

- Chamomile (Matricaria chamomilla): Chamomile is a gentle herb known for its calming properties. It can help reduce anxiety and promote better sleep. Whether consumed as a tea or used in aromatherapy, chamomile offers a natural and soothing remedy for stress-related symptoms.

Rituals and Practices

Traditional tribal cultures often incorporate unique rituals and practices into their daily lives to promote emotional well-being. These include:

- Smudging: Smudging involves burning sacred herbs, such as sage or cedar, to cleanse the energy and create a sense of purification. This practice is believed to clear negative energy and promote emotional balance.

- Using Salt, Oils, and Incense: Another method of cleansing in traditional tribal cultures is the use of salt, oils, and incense. Salt is often used to create a protective barrier and cleanse negative energy from a space. Oils, such as essential oils, can be used for aromatherapy to promote relaxation and emotional well-being. Incense is burned to purify the air and create a sacred atmosphere. These practices can be incorporated into daily rituals or ceremonies to enhance emotional well-being and promote a sense of harmony.

- Chanting: Chanting is another common practice in traditional tribal cultures. It involves repetitive vocalization of sacred words or sounds. Chanting is believed to have a calming effect on the mind and can help promote focus, relaxation, and spiritual connection. You can chant affirmations of tribal melodies that resonate with you.

As we've seen, exploring ancient tribal remedies for emotional wellness can provide valuable insights into alternative approaches to emotional well-being. While these remedies have shown effectiveness, it is important to exercise caution and consult with healthcare professionals, especially when using them in conjunction with other medications or treatments. By embracing the wisdom of traditional tribal approaches, women can expand their toolkit for managing emotional well-being and find a path towards greater balance and harmony in their lives.

A Special Note from the Author

Dear Reader,

As you pause here at the midpoint of our journey together, I hope you've found the pages so far to be enlightening and enjoyable. If this book has touched you, sparked new thoughts, or offered valuable insights, I have a small favor to ask.

Would you consider leaving a review?

Your thoughts and experiences matter immensely. By sharing a review, you not only support me as an author but also guide others who could benefit from this book. Your words can illuminate the path for someone else seeking the insights and knowledge you've discovered.

If you don't have time for a review, please take just a brief moment to leave a star rating if you find this book to be valuable.

Thank you for being a part of this story. Your voice can make a profound difference.

Warm regards,

Nya Love

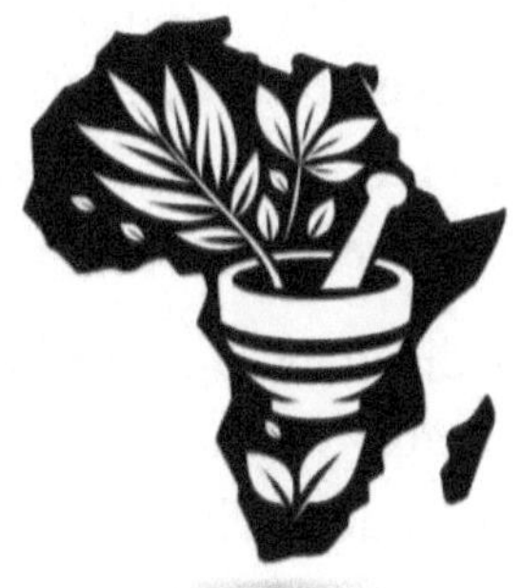

Chapter 6
Holistic Body Care with Ancestral Cures

The Divine Feminine is the portal for holistic health.

As African American Women living in a society that often emphasizes external beauty standards and places immense pressure on individuals to conform, it is crucial to reconnect with our inner selves and embrace the Divine Feminine within.

We've made it to Chapter 6 of our book, over half way there! In this chapter we will be merging the knowledge of Divine Feminine energy which we have gained with ancestral remedies and holistic body care.

This chapter delves deep into the practices and principles that can empower women to nurture themselves, prioritize self-care, and develop a positive body image. By drawing inspiration from ancestral wisdom and embracing holistic approaches, we can unlock the secrets to a more fulfilling and harmonious relationship with our bodies. We will also explore traditional methods of body care and maintenance, including how to create homemade beauty and skincare products, and emphasize the benefits of natural remedies for physical well-being.

Throughout these pages, we will explore the profound connection between embracing the Divine Feminine and cultivating self-compassion. We will uncover the transformative power of ancestral cures and rituals that have been passed down through generations, offering us a unique perspective on holistic body care.

On this journey of self-discovery, exploring the ancient wisdom that lies within our ancestral heritage is a continuous endeavor. Through the exploration of these practices and principles, we will learn to honor our bodies, embrace our uniqueness, and foster a deep sense of self-love and acceptance.

Let us dive right into the transformative world of self-compassion and self-love, where the Divine Feminine awaits to guide us towards a more harmonious and fulfilling existence.

Cultivating Self-Compassion Through the Lens of the Divine Feminine

Self-Compassion: Nurturing Personal Growth and Well-Being

Self-compassion, a concept rooted in mindfulness and self-kindness, plays a pivotal role in fostering personal growth and enhancing overall well-being. It involves treating oneself with the same warmth, understanding, and support that one would offer to a close friend facing challenges or setbacks. By cultivating self-compassion, individuals can develop a healthier relationship with themselves, leading to increased resilience, improved mental health, and a greater sense of fulfillment.

At its core, self-compassion involves acknowledging and accepting one's own imperfections and limitations without judgment or self-criticism. Rather than berating oneself for mistakes or perceived shortcomings, self-compassion encourages individuals to embrace their humanity and respond with kindness and understanding. This compassionate mindset allows for greater self-acceptance and a more positive outlook on life.

One of the key benefits of self-compassion is its ability to promote personal growth. When humans approach their own struggles and failures with self-compassion, they create a safe space for learning and growth. Instead of being paralyzed by self-doubt or fear of failure, they can view setbacks as opportunities for growth and development. This mindset shift fosters resilience and encourages us to persevere in the face of challenges, ultimately leading to personal growth and achievement.

Moreover, self-compassion is closely linked to improved mental health and well-being. Research has shown that those who practice self-compassion experience lower levels of anxiety, depression, and stress. By offering themselves kindness and understanding, they develop a greater sense of emotional well-being and inner peace. Self-compassion also helps individuals cultivate a positive self-image, fostering self-esteem and self-worth.

By treating yourself with kindness, understanding, and acceptance, you can foster resilience, enhance mental health, and cultivate a positive self-image. Embracing self-compassion allows us women to navigate life's challenges with grace and self-assurance, leading to a more fulfilling and meaningful existence.

Title: Cultivating Self-Compassion through the Lens of the Divine Feminine

In a world that often emphasizes achievement, productivity, and self-criticism, cultivating self-compassion has become essential for our well-being. Embracing the qualities associated with the Divine Feminine offers a nurturing and compassionate framework for women to develop self-compassion. In this section we will explore how connecting with the Divine Feminine can provide practical techniques and exercises to foster self-compassion.

Some ways to understand the Divine Feminine intimately include:

- Embracing Vulnerability: Vulnerability is a key aspect of self-compassion. By embracing vulnerability, we acknowledge our imperfections and allow ourselves to be seen authentically. The Divine Feminine encourages us to embrace vulnerability as a strength, fostering self-compassion. One practical technique is to engage in journaling, allowing ourselves to express our emotions and thoughts without judgment.

- Cultivating Self-Love: Self-love is an integral part of self-compassion. The Divine Feminine teaches us to love ourselves unconditionally, just as we would love others. To cultivate self-love, we can practice affirmations and positive self-talk. Affirmations such as "I am worthy of love and compassion" can help rewire negative self-perceptions and foster a compassionate mindset.

- Connecting with Nature: Nature is a powerful teacher of compassion and interconnectedness. The Divine Feminine is deeply intertwined with the natural world. Spending time in nature, whether it's taking a walk in the park or sitting by a serene lake, can help us reconnect with our own inner nature and cultivate self-compassion. Engaging in grounding exercises, such as barefoot walking or mindful breathing, can enhance this connection.

- ways

- Embodying Forgiveness: Forgiveness is a transformative practice that allows us to release self-judgment and embrace self-compassion. The Divine Feminine encourages us to embody forgiveness towards ourselves and others. One technique is to write a forgiveness letter to ourselves, acknowledging past mistakes and offering compassion and understanding. This exercise can help us let go of self-blame and cultivate self-compassion.

- Cultivating Intuition: Intuition is a powerful tool for self-compassion. The Divine Feminine emphasizes the importance of listening to our inner wisdom and trusting our instincts. To cultivate intuition, we can engage in mindfulness practices, such as meditation or body scans, to quiet the mind and connect with our inner guidance. Trusting our intuition allows us to make choices aligned with self-compassion.

- Practicing Self-Care: Self-care is an essential aspect of self-compassion. The Divine Feminine reminds us to prioritize our well-being and nourish ourselves physically, emotionally, and spiritually. Engaging in activities that bring joy and relaxation, such as taking a bath, practicing yoga, or engaging in creative pursuits, can help us replenish our energy and cultivate self-compassion.

Cultivating self-compassion through the lens of the Divine Feminine offers a nurturing and compassionate framework for women seeking to embrace their own worthiness and well-being. Two Important aspects of compassion—self-care and self-love—can be a little difficult to understand. Let's break them both down

Practicing Self-Care as an Act of Self-Love

This section will delve into the significance of self-care in maintaining physical, emotional, and spiritual well-being.I will highlight the connection between self-care and self-love, emphasizing how prioritizing self-care is an act of love towards oneself.

The section will offer various self-care practices and rituals that can be incorporated into daily life, drawing inspiration from the energy of the Divine Feminine.

Self-care is a fundamental aspect of maintaining overall well-being. It encompasses various practices and activities that prioritize and nurture our physical, emotional, and spiritual health. Let's explore the significance of self-care and how it contributes to our overall well-being.

Physical Well-Being

Self-care plays a crucial role in maintaining our physical health. Engaging in regular exercise, eating a balanced diet, and getting enough rest are essential components of self-care. By prioritizing physical well-being, we can enhance our energy levels, improve our immune system, and reduce the risk of chronic illnesses. Additionally, self-care practices such as regular check-ups and preventive healthcare measures contribute to early detection and effective management of potential health issues.

Emotional Well-Being

Taking care of our emotional well-being is equally important. Self-care practices such as mindfulness, meditation, and journaling allow us to connect with our emotions, process them, and develop emotional resilience. Engaging in activities that bring us joy, spending time with loved ones, and setting healthy boundaries also contribute to emotional well-being. By practicing self-care, we can reduce stress, manage anxiety and depression, and cultivate a positive mindset.

Spiritual Well-Being

Nurturing our spiritual well-being is an integral part of self-care. This involves connecting with our inner selves, exploring our values and beliefs, and finding meaning and purpose in life. Engaging in practices such as prayer, meditation, or spending time in nature can help us cultivate a sense of spirituality. By prioritizing our spiritual well-being, we can experience a greater sense of peace, fulfillment, and connection to something larger than ourselves.

It is important to recognize that physical, emotional, and spiritual well-being are interconnected. Neglecting one aspect can have a detrimental impact on the others. For example, chronic stress can lead to physical ailments and emotional distress. By practicing self-care holistically, we can create a harmonious balance between these dimensions of well-being, leading to a more fulfilling and meaningful life.

Self-care is not a luxury but a necessity for maintaining physical, emotional, and spiritual well-being as a woman. By prioritizing self-care practices, we can enhance our overall quality of life, improve our relationships, and cultivate a greater sense of self-awareness and fulfillment. Self-care is an ongoing journey that requires conscious effort and commitment.

Self-care and self-love are two intertwined concepts that play a crucial role in our overall well-being. While self-care refers to the intentional actions we take to nurture our physical, mental, and emotional health, self-love is the deep appreciation and acceptance of oneself. These two concepts go hand in hand, as prioritizing self-care is, in essence, an act of love towards oneself.

At the core of self-care lies the understanding that we are deserving of love, care, and attention. By engaging in self-care practices, we acknowledge our worth and prioritize our own needs. This act of prioritization is an act of self-love. When we make time for activities that bring us joy, rest, and rejuvenation, we are sending a powerful message to ourselves that we matter and that our well-being is important.

Self-care acts as a foundation for cultivating self-love. When we consistently engage in self-care practices, we develop a deeper connection with ourselves. We become more attuned to our needs, desires, and boundaries. This heightened self-awareness allows us to make choices that align with our values and promote our overall happiness and fulfillment.

Moreover, self-care acts as a buffer against stress and burnout. When we neglect our own well-being, we become more susceptible to physical and emotional exhaustion. By prioritizing self-care, we replenish our energy reserves and build resilience. This, in turn, strengthens our self-love, as we recognize the importance of taking care of ourselves in order to show up fully in our lives and relationships.

Additionally, self-care fosters a positive self-image and boosts self-esteem. When we engage in activities that promote self-care, such as exercise, healthy eating, or engaging in hobbies we enjoy, we feel a sense of accomplishment and pride. These positive experiences contribute to a healthier self-perception and reinforce our self-love.

IBy embracing self-care practices, we cultivate self-love, leading to a more fulfilling and balanced life. Remember, taking care of yourself is not selfish; it is an essential act of self-love that allows you to thrive and be the best version of yourself.

Embracing the Divine Feminine: Nurturing Self-Care Practices for Daily Life

It is crucial to prioritize self-care and reconnect with our inner selves In today's world. Drawing inspiration from the energy of the Divine Feminine, we can cultivate a deeper sense of well-being and balance in our daily lives. This section explores various self-care practices and rituals that can be incorporated into our routines, allowing us to honor and embrace our feminine essence.

1. Mindful Morning Rituals: To start the day on a positive note, consider incorporating mindful morning rituals. Begin by setting aside a few moments for meditation or deep breathing exercises. This helps to calm the mind, reduce stress, and set intentions for the day ahead. You can follow this with gentle stretching or yoga to awaken the body and promote flexibility. Finally, nourish yourself with a nutritious breakfast, savoring each bite mindfully. You can also incorporate affirmations during your intention setting practice.

2. Sacred Bathing: Bathing can be transformed into a sacred ritual by infusing it with the energy of the Divine Feminine. Create a serene ambiance in your bathroom with soft lighting, soothing music, and aromatic candles. Add a few drops of essential oils, such as lavender or rose, to your bathwater. As you soak, visualize the water cleansing and rejuvenating your body, mind, and spirit. Allow yourself to fully relax and let go of any tension or negativity.

3. Journaling and Reflection: As I've previously noted, writing can be a powerful tool for self-discovery and self-expression. Set aside time each day to journal your thoughts, feelings, and experiences. This practice allows you to connect with your

innermost desires, fears, and aspirations. Reflect on your journey, celebrate your achievements, and explore areas for growth. Embrace the wisdom of the Divine Feminine as you pour your heart onto the pages, finding clarity and insight along the way. Journaling for 20 minutes a day has been proven to

4. Mindful Cooking: Spending time in the kitchen is a wonderful way to engage with your creativity and nourish your body. Try experimenting with new recipes and ingredients, and savor the process of preparing a delicious meal. Engage your senses by observing the colors, aromas, and flavors that come together in the culinary world. Even if you're not good at cooking, and the outcome isn't so spectacular, mindful cooking and baking are deeply therapeutic practices; when you're not under pressure that is.

5. Allow yourself to be present in the moment, grounding yourself and finding solace in the embrace of Mother Earth.

6. Creative Expression: Embrace your creative side as a form of self-care. Engage in activities that bring you joy and allow you to express yourself authentically. This could include painting, writing poetry, dancing, singing, or playing a musical instrument. Let go of any self-judgment and allow your creativity to flow freely. By nurturing your creative spirit, you tap into the Divine Feminine's energy of creation and bring more beauty into your life.

Affirmations to Start the Day With DF Self-Love

- "I am worthy of love, happiness, and abundance in all areas of my life."

- "I embrace my unique qualities and celebrate the woman I am becoming."

- "I prioritize self-care and make time for activities that nourish my mind, body, and soul."

- "I release any negative thoughts or limiting beliefs that no longer serve me."

- "I am grateful for the blessings in my life and open to receiving more."

- "I trust my intuition and make decisions that align with my highest good."

- "I attract positive and supportive relationships that uplift and inspire me."

- "I am confident in my abilities and trust in my own inner strength."

- "I let go of comparison and embrace my own journey, knowing that I am enough."

- "I am deserving of success and I take inspired action towards my goals."

Incorporating self-care practices and rituals inspired by the Divine Feminine can have a profound impact on our overall well-being. By prioritizing our self-care, we honor our feminine essence and create a harmonious balance in our lives.

Prioritizing self-care is an act of love towards oneself. It is important to recognize that physical, emotional, and spiritual well-being are interconnected. Neglecting one aspect can have a detrimental impact on the others. For example, chronic stress can lead to physical ailments and emotional distress. By practicing self-care holistically, we can create a harmonious balance between these dimensions of well-being, leading to a more fulfilling and meaningful life.

Self-care is not a luxury but a necessity for maintaining physical, emotional, and spiritual well-being as a woman. By prioritizing self-care practices, we can enhance our overall quality of life, improve our relationships, and cultivate a greater sense of self-awareness and fulfillment. Self-care is an ongoing journey that requires conscious effort and commitment. When we love ourselves, we are honoring our divine feminine essence.

Fostering a Positive Body Image and Nurturing the Self

In today's society, the pressure to conform to societal standards of beauty and the constant bombardment of unrealistic body ideals can have a detrimental impact on our body image and self-worth. This section aims to delve into the profound influence of societal standards and cultural conditioning on body image perceptions. Furthermore, it will explore how embracing the Divine Feminine can empower individuals to challenge and overcome negative body image perceptions. Finally, we will provide practical tools and techniques for nurturing and embracing the self, promoting self-acceptance, and fostering a positive body image.

Impact of Societal Standards and Cultural Conditioning

Societal standards of beauty, perpetuated by media, advertising, and social platforms, often promote a narrow and unrealistic ideal of what is considered attractive. This constant exposure to unattainable beauty standards can lead to feelings of inadequacy, low self-esteem, and negative body image. Moreover, cultural conditioning plays a significant role in shaping our perceptions of beauty, as different cultures may have varying ideals and expectations. It is crucial to recognize the influence of these external factors and understand how they can impact our self-perception.

By embracing DF qualities, women can challenge societal norms and redefine their own standards of beauty. Embracing the Divine Feminine involves recognizing and celebrating the uniqueness and inherent beauty of every individual, regardless of societal expectations. This shift in perspective allows for a more inclusive and empowering approach to body image.

Challenging Negative Body Image Perceptions

To overcome negative body image perceptions, it is essential to cultivate self-compassion and challenge negative self-talk. This can be achieved through practices such as affirmations, mindfulness, and self-reflection. Mindfulness helps you become aware of your thoughts and emotions without judgment, allowing you to detach from negative body image narratives. Affirmations, such as repeating positive statements about oneself, can help rewire negative thought patterns and promote self-acceptance. Self-reflection encourages individuals to explore the root causes of their negative body image and develop strategies to address them.

Promoting self-acceptance and fostering a positive body image requires a holistic approach. Here are some practical tools and techniques to nurture and embrace yourself fully:

- Engage in activities that promote self-care, such as exercise, healthy eating, and getting enough rest. Taking care of your physical and mental well-being can positively impact your body image.

- Surround yourself with positive influences. These include supportive and body-positive individuals who celebrate diversity and promote self-acceptance. Limit exposure to media that perpetuates unrealistic beauty standards.

- Cultivate gratitude for your body and its capabilities. Focus on what your body can do rather than how it looks. Express gratitude for the unique qualities that make you who you are.

- Seek Professional Help. If negative body image persists and significantly impacts your well-being, consider seeking support from a therapist or counselor who specializes in body image issues.

Fostering a positive body image and nurturing oneself is a journey that requires self-reflection, self-compassion, and a shift in perspective. By challenging societal standards, embracing the Divine Feminine, and utilizing practical tools and techniques, we can overcome negative body image perceptions and cultivate a positive relationship with our bodies. Remember, true beauty lies in embracing and celebrating our unique selves.

Learning how to Create Homemade Beauty and Skincare Products

Body holistic care can also be fun and relaxing. It is not always hard work and releasing limiting conditioning.

Creating your own homemade beauty and skincare products can be a rewarding and empowering experience. Not only do you have control over the ingredients you use, but you also have the opportunity to tap into ancestral recipes that have been passed down through generations.

In this final section of the chapter, I will provide step-by-step guidance on how to create natural, homemade beauty and skincare products that leave you feeling pampered and rejuvenated.

Creating Nourishing and Effective Skincare Products with Natural Ingredients

By combining fruits, herbs, and essential oils, you can create nourishing and effective products that cater to your specific skincare needs.

Facial Masks:

Avocado and Honey Mask:

- Mash half an avocado and mix it with one tablespoon of honey.

- Apply the mixture to your face and leave it on for 15-20 minutes.

- Rinse off with warm water to reveal hydrated and glowing skin.

- This Avocado and Honey Mask helps to hydrate and nourish the skin, leaving it looking radiant and glowing.

Oatmeal and Yogurt Mask:

- Mix two tablespoons of oatmeal with one tablespoon of yogurt.

- Apply the mixture to your face and gently massage in circular motions.

- Leave it on for 10-15 minutes and rinse off with lukewarm water.

- This mask helps to exfoliate and soothe the skin.

Hair Treatments:

Coconut Oil and Honey Hair Mask:

- Mix two tablespoons of coconut oil with one tablespoon of honey.

- Apply the mixture to damp hair, focusing on the ends.

- Leave it on for 30 minutes to an hour, then rinse thoroughly.

- This mask helps to nourish and moisturize dry and damaged hair.

Banana and Olive Oil Hair Mask:

- Mash one ripe banana and mix it with two tablespoons of olive oil.

- Apply the mixture to your hair, starting from the roots to the ends.

- Leave it on for 30 minutes, then wash your hair as usual.

- This mask helps to add shine and improve hair elasticity.

Body Oils:

Lavender and Almond Oil Blend:

- Mix five drops of lavender essential oil with two tablespoons of almond oil.

- Massage the oil blend onto your body after a shower or bath.

- This blend helps to relax the mind and nourish the skin.

Citrus and Jojoba Oil Blend:

- Mix five drops of citrus essential oil (such as orange or lemon) with two tablespoons of jojoba oil.

- Apply the oil blend to your body, focusing on dry areas.

- This blend helps to invigorate and moisturize the skin.

By combining natural ingredients like fruits, herbs, and essential oils, you can create nourishing and effective skincare products at home. Experiment with different recipes and find what works best for your specific skincare needs. Enjoy the benefits of nature's bounty and pamper yourself or loved ones with these homemade treatments.

There are numerous benefits of using homemade products that are free from harmful chemicals and additives. Commercial beauty and skincare products often contain synthetic ingredients that can be harsh on the skin and may have long-term negative effects. By creating your own products, you can ensure that you are using only natural and organic ingredients that are gentle and beneficial for your skin.

With regular practice, you can gain the knowledge and confidence to create your own homemade beauty and skincare products. Whether you are looking to treat yourself or share your creations with others, this is a journey of natural self-care and beauty. It is also great creative expression and fun!

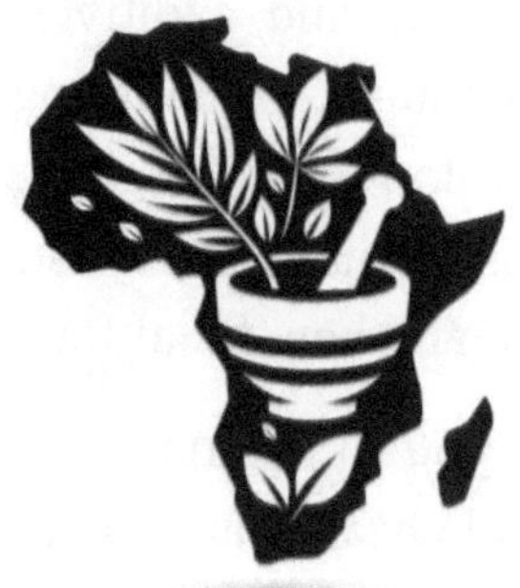

Chapter 7
Spiritual Healing with Ancestral Wisdom

Of course, a book about holistic health for women had to have a chapter delving into spiritual healing and growth. In the upcoming pages, we will explore the importance of connecting with ancestral knowledge and traditions for our spiritual well-being.

We will delve into various spiritual practices and rituals from different cultures worldwide. Through this exploration, we will gain insights on cultivating a personal spiritual practice rooted in the wisdom of our ancestors. Get ready to discover ancient parts of yourself and find spiritual enlightenment.

Understanding the Role of Spirituality in Overall Well-being

Spirituality plays a significant role in achieving holistic well-being. It encompasses a deep connection with oneself, others, and the universe, providing a sense of purpose, meaning, and fulfillment in life. While physical and mental health are crucial, spirituality adds another dimension to our well-being.

One of the key aspects of spirituality is the exploration of our inner selves. It involves self-reflection, introspection, and understanding our values, beliefs, and purpose in life. By delving into our spiritual nature, we gain a deeper understanding of ourselves, which can lead to increased self-acceptance and self-love.

Spirituality also fosters a sense of interconnectedness with others and the world around us. It encourages empathy, compassion, and a desire to contribute positively to society. When we recognize that we are part of something greater than ourselves, it brings a sense of unity and belonging.

Moreover, spirituality provides solace and support during challenging times. It offers a source of strength, hope, and resilience, enabling individuals to navigate through life's difficulties with grace and courage. Spiritual practices such as meditation, prayer, or mindfulness can help reduce stress, promote relaxation, and enhance overall well-being.

All-in-all, spirituality is an integral component of overall well-being. It nurtures our inner selves, strengthens our connections with others, and provides guidance and support in our journey through life. By acknowledging and embracing spirituality, we can achieve a more balanced and fulfilling existence.

Spirituality is a deeply personal and subjective experience that can provide women with a profound sense of purpose, meaning, and connectedness to themselves, others, and the world. It goes beyond religious beliefs and practices, encompassing a broader understanding of the human experience and our place in the universe.

Spirituality and its Role in Providing Purpose, Meaning, and Connectedness

At its core, spirituality allows individuals to introspect and explore, seeking answers to life's fundamental questions. It provides a framework for understanding the deeper meaning and purpose behind our existence, beyond the materialistic pursuits of everyday life. Through spiritual practices such as meditation, prayer, or mindfulness, individuals can cultivate a sense of inner peace, clarity, and self-awareness.

Spirituality also fosters a sense of connectedness to others. It recognizes the inherent interconnectedness of all living beings and promotes empathy, compassion, and love towards others. By acknowledging our shared humanity, spirituality encourages individuals to treat others with kindness, respect, and understanding. This interconnectedness extends beyond human relationships to include a sense of reverence and respect for the natural world, fostering a deep connection to the environment and all living creatures.

Moreover, spirituality can provide women with a sense of purpose. It helps individuals align their actions and values with a higher sense of meaning and significance. By connecting with our inner values and beliefs, we can find a sense of direction and fulfillment in their lives. This sense of purpose can guide decision-making, inspire personal growth, and contribute to a greater sense of overall well-being.

Spirituality plays a significant role in promoting overall well-being, encompassing mental, emotional, and physical aspects of life. It offers a unique perspective that goes beyond the materialistic world, focusing on inner growth, connection, and finding meaning in life. In this section, we will delve into how spirituality can contribute to enhancing well-being and fostering balance and harmony in all aspects of life.

Mental well-being is greatly influenced by spirituality. Engaging in spiritual practices such as meditation, mindfulness, or prayer can help calm the mind, reduce stress, and enhance mental clarity. By connecting with a higher power or a sense of purpose, individuals often find solace and a sense of inner peace, which positively impacts their mental state.

Emotional well-being is closely intertwined with spirituality. Exploring one's spirituality allows individuals to tap into their emotions, understand their feelings, and develop a deeper sense of self-awareness. This self-reflection and introspection can lead to emotional healing, personal growth, and the ability to navigate life's challenges with resilience and grace.

Physical well-being can also be influenced by spirituality. Many spiritual practices emphasize the importance of taking care of the body as a temple. Engaging in activities such as yoga, tai chi, or mindful movement not only promote physical fitness but also cultivate a sense of connection between the body, mind, and spirit. This holistic approach to health can lead to increased vitality, reduced stress-related ailments, and a greater sense of overall well-being.

Furthermore, spirituality provides a framework for living a balanced and harmonious life. It encourages individuals to align their actions and values with their spiritual beliefs, fostering a sense of purpose, integrity, and ethical behavior. This alignment promotes a sense of inner harmony and fulfillment, which positively impacts relationships, work-life balance, and overall life satisfaction.

Exploring Spiritual Practices and Rituals from Different Cultures

As a fundamental aspect of human existence, spirituality manifests in various forms across different cultures worldwide. This section aims to look at the rich tapestry of spiritual practices and rituals found within various cultures. By exploring these diverse traditions, we can gain a deeper understanding of the human quest for connection, meaning, and transcendence.

African Spiritual Practices and Rituals

Africa is a continent known for its vibrant and diverse spiritual traditions. From the ancient Egyptian civilization to the indigenous tribes of sub-Saharan Africa, spiritual practices and rituals play a central role in daily life. For instance, in Yoruba culture, the Ifa divination system is used to communicate with the deities and ancestors, seeking guidance and wisdom. Similarly, in the Akan tradition, the pouring of libations is a ritual act of honoring and connecting with the spirits of the ancestors.

African American Spiritual Practices and Rituals

The African diaspora brought forth a unique blend of African and American cultural elements, resulting in distinctive spiritual practices among African Americans. One prominent example is the tradition of Hoodoo, which combines African folk magic, Native American herbalism, and Christian elements. Hoodoo practitioners engage in rituals involving the use of herbs, candles, and spiritual baths to address various needs, such as protection, love, and prosperity. This blend is the central focus of many of the practices in this book.

Tribal and Native Spiritual Practices and Rituals

Indigenous cultures around the world have deep-rooted spiritual practices and rituals that are intimately connected to their relationship with nature and the land. Native American tribes, for instance, engage in sacred ceremonies like the Sun Dance, Sweat Lodge, and Vision Quest, which serve as transformative experiences and opportunities for spiritual growth. These rituals often involve fasting, prayer, and communal participation, fostering a sense of unity and connection with the natural world. We will explore a few of these rituals in depth later on in the book.

It is easy to see how these spiritual practices tie in with healing and holistic well-being.

Cross-Cultural Influences and Adaptations

It is important to note that spiritual practices and rituals are not static; they evolve and adapt over time. Cultural exchange and globalization have led to the blending of traditions, resulting in new syncretic practices. For example, Santeria, a religion that originated in Cuba, combines elements of Yoruba spirituality with Catholicism. This fusion reflects the resilience and adaptability of spiritual practices as they navigate changing social and cultural landscapes.

Exploring spiritual practices and rituals from different cultures, particularly within African, African American, and tribal/native communities, reveals the profound diversity and richness of human spiritual expression and the interconnected nature of existence. These practices serve as a testament to the universal human longing for connection, meaning, and transcendence. There are a number of practices that can fall under these traditions, unique to each woman's chosen spiritual journey.

Nurturing Spiritual Healing and Growth

Spiritual practices have been an integral part of human existence for centuries, serving as pathways to connect with the divine, seek inner peace, and promote spiritual healing and growth. In order to take charge of your spiritual journey, it is important to explore various spiritual practices, all the while shedding light on their significance and the cultural and historical context that surrounds them. By delving into these practices, you can gain a deeper understanding of their purpose and foster appreciation and respect for the ancestral wisdom they embody.

Though mindfulness-based meditation has become the most popular narrative in the mainstream, primarily for mental and emotional well-being, meditation is originally a spiritual practice. As you now know, meditation, a practice rooted in ancient traditions, involves quieting the mind and turning inward. This can achieve a state of deep relaxation, clear introspection, self-care, and heightened awareness.

With the intent of spiritual gain and connection, meditation allows women to cultivate a sense of inner peace, clarity, and self-discovery. More importantly, the identity based ego self dissolves during meditation, and the meditator becomes connected with the oneness of existence-the direct expression of divine energy. By focusing on the breath or a specific mantra, practitioners can transcend the limitations of the physical world and tap into the vast realm of spiritual consciousness.

Another widely practiced spiritual tradition is Prayer. Prayer serves as a means of communication with the divine. It is a deeply personal and heartfelt expression of cosmic trust, gratitude, and, in some cases, supplication. Through prayer, women seek solace, guidance, and spiritual connection, finding comfort in the belief that their words are heard and answered by a higher power. Across cultures and religions, prayer has been a source of strength and a catalyst for spiritual healing and growth.

Chanting, often accompanied by rhythmic music or repetitive vocalizations, is a practice that transcends language barriers and taps into the power of sound vibrations. Chants, whether in the form of mantras, hymns, or sacred verses, have been used for centuries to invoke spiritual energies, elevate consciousness, and create a harmonious connection between the individual and the divine. Chanting not only promotes spiritual healing but also fosters a sense of unity and collective consciousness among participants.

Dance, in its various forms, has long been recognized as a powerful medium for spiritual expression and transformation. From the whirling dervishes of Sufism to the ecstatic dances of indigenous cultures, movement becomes a conduit for connecting with the divine. Through dance, individuals can transcend the limitations of the physical body, enter a state of ecstatic bliss, and experience a profound sense of unity with the universe.

Sacred ceremonies, deeply rooted in cultural and historical contexts, are rituals that honor and celebrate the sacred. These ceremonies often involve specific rites, symbols, and practices passed down through generations. They serve as powerful vehicles for spiritual healing and growth, providing a sense of belonging, connection, and reverence for the divine and the interconnectedness of all beings.

You can begin embracing any of these practices as tools for personal growth, spiritual healing, and foster a greater connection with the Divine Feminine.

By exploring these spiritual practices and understanding their cultural and historical significance, you can develop a deeper appreciation for the wisdom and traditions of your ancestors. You can embrace these practices as tools for personal growth, spiritual healing, and fostering a greater connection with the divine. In doing so, the fruits of self-discovery, inner peace, and spiritual enlightenment are revealed.

Creating Your Personal Spiritual Practice Rooted in Ancestral Traditions

Learning how to create a personal spiritual practice rooted in ancestral traditions is a transformative journey that can deeply enrich our lives. As we embark on this path, it is important to guide readers in developing their own unique practice that resonates with their individual preferences and beliefs.

To begin, incorporating ancestral wisdom into our daily lives can be achieved through simple yet meaningful rituals. Whether it's lighting a candle, offering gratitude to our ancestors, or engaging in meditation, these practices connect us to our roots and provide a sense of grounding and connection.

Honoring traditions is another vital aspect of our personal spiritual practice. By learning about our ancestral customs, rituals, and celebrations, we can infuse our lives with the wisdom and teachings of those who came before us. This not only fosters a deeper understanding of our heritage but also strengthens our connection to our lineage.

Adapting practices to suit our individual preferences and beliefs is essential in creating a personal spiritual practice. We are all unique beings with diverse experiences and perspectives. Therefore, it is crucial to explore different modalities, such as prayer, chanting, or energy work, and find what resonates with us on a deep level.

Establishing a consistent spiritual practice offers numerous benefits. It provides a sacred space for self-reflection, introspection, and personal growth. Through regular engagement with our ancestral traditions, we can cultivate a sense of inner peace, clarity, and spiritual well-being. This practice becomes a source of strength and guidance, supporting us in navigating life's challenges and fostering a deeper connection to ourselves and the world around us.

By embarking on the journey of creating a personal spiritual practice rooted in ancestral traditions, readers have the opportunity to experience transformative self-discovery and growth. It is my deepest hope that so far this guide book has inspired and empowered you to embrace your heritage, honor your ancestors, and cultivate a holistic practice that nourishes your soul, mind, heart, and body.

In the next chapter, we will look further into Incorporating Ancestral Remedies into Daily Life.

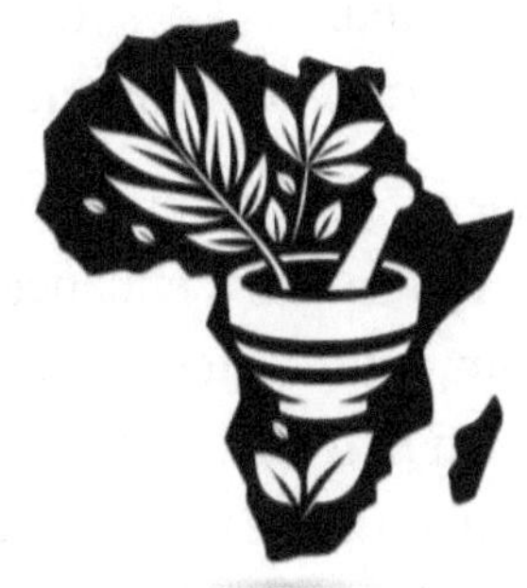

Chapter 8
Incorporating Ancestral Remedies into Daily Life

I'm proud of you for coming so far on your journey toward holistic health and ancestral healing. We only have two chapters left in this guidebook, and most of your devoted work toward self-love and improvement has already begun.

In this chapter, we delve into the realm of ancestral remedies and their integration into our daily routines for enhanced well-being. As the real journey has only just begun, I will offer practical guidance, empowering you to create a self-care plan that embraces the wisdom of our ancestors. By incorporating ancestral remedies into your life, you can unlock a wealth of benefits for your physical, mental, and emotional health.

We will explore the art of crafting rituals and habits that nurture your well-being in the long run. These rituals, rooted in ancient wisdom, have the power to restore balance and harmony to your life. Rituals are repetitive tasks that are performed with the intention of creating a sense of connection and meaning. Moreover, we will address the challenges and obstacles that may arise when implementing ancestral remedies, equipping you with strategies to overcome them.

It's time to navigate the path to improved well-being through the integration of ancestral remedies. Let's discover the transformative potential of honoring our heritage and embracing our healing practices.

In this chapter, we delve into the realm of ancestral remedies and their integration into our daily routines for enhanced well-being. As the real journey has only just begun, I will offer practical guidance, empowering you to create a self-care plan that embraces the wisdom of our ancestors. By incorporating ancestral remedies into your life, you can unlock a wealth of benefits for your physical, mental, and emotional health.

We will explore the art of crafting rituals and habits that nurture your well-being in the long run. These rituals, rooted in ancient wisdom, have the power to restore balance and harmony to your life. Rituals are repetitive tasks that are performed with the intention of creating a sense of connection and meaning. Moreover, we will address the challenges and obstacles that may arise when implementing ancestral remedies, equipping you with strategies to overcome them.

It's time to navigate the path to improved well-being through the integration of ancestral remedies. Let's discover the transformative potential of honoring our heritage and embracing our healing practices.

Rituals are simply repetitive tasks for connection and meaning.

"'Creating a self-care plan that incorporates ancestral remedies'"

In today's fast-paced world, self-care has become more important than ever. Taking care of ourselves is crucial for maintaining physical, mental, and emotional well-being. While there are countless modern self-care practices available, incorporating ancestral remedies, including those in this book, into our self-care routines can provide a unique and powerful connection to our roots.

When it comes to creating a comprehensive self-care plan, it is important to consider the incorporation of ancestral remedies. These practices and their wisdom have stood the test of time.

One of the key aspects of incorporating ancestral remedies into a self-care plan is the identification of specific remedies that align with individual needs and goals. Each person is unique, and their self-care requirements can vary greatly. By understanding our specific needs and goals, we can identify the ancestral remedies that can support and nourish us in a holistic way.

To begin the process, it is important to reflect on our heritage and cultural background. Exploring the traditions and practices of our ancestors can reveal valuable insights into the healing remedies that have been passed down through generations. By understanding our roots, we can tap into a rich source of knowledge and wisdom that can guide us in creating a self-care plan that is aligned with our heritage.

Once we have gained an understanding of our ancestral heritage, we can then explore the various ancestral remedies that resonate with us. This can involve researching traditional healing practices, consulting with knowledgeable individuals like elders or cultural experts, and experimenting with different remedies to find what works best for us.

Additionally, it is important to consider the practical aspects of incorporating ancestral remedies into our self-care routine. This may involve sourcing natural ingredients, learning how to prepare remedies, and creating a sustainable and consistent practice. It is essential to approach ancestral remedies with respect and reverence, honoring the traditions and wisdom that they carry.

Incorporating ancestral remedies into a self-care plan offers numerous benefits. These remedies are often deeply rooted in nature and promote a more holistic approach to well-being. They can provide a sense of connection to our heritage and ancestors, fostering a deeper understanding of our cultural identity. By incorporating these remedies into our daily lives, we can cultivate a greater sense of balance, rejuvenation, and overall well-being.

All-in-all, creating a self-care plan that incorporates ancestral remedies is a meaningful way to honor our heritage and take care of ourselves holistically. By identifying specific remedies that align with our individual needs and goals, and approaching them with respect and reverence, we can tap into a wealth of ancestral wisdom and nourish ourselves in a profound way.

Let us embrace our roots and embrace the power of ancestral remedies in our self-care journeys.

You may be wondering how to seamlessly integrate these unique ancestral remedies into your daily routines, allowing you to establish a sustainable self-care practice. By following the guidance provided in this book, you can unlock the full potential of these remedies and experience their transformative benefits.

To begin, start by identifying the specific ancestral remedies that resonate with you the most. Whether it's herbal teas, essential oils, or traditional healing practices, choose the remedies that align with your personal needs and preferences. This will ensure that your self-care practice feels authentic and tailored to your unique journey.

Once you have identified your preferred remedies, incorporate them into your daily routines in a way that feels natural and effortless. For example, if you enjoy starting your day with a calming cup of herbal tea, make it a ritual by setting aside a few moments each morning to prepare and savor your brew. This simple act of mindfulness can help you cultivate a sense of tranquility and set a positive tone for the day ahead.

Additionally, consider integrating these remedies into existing self-care practices. For instance, if you already have a skincare routine, explore the use of natural ingredients and ancestral beauty secrets to enhance the nourishing effects on your skin. This can include incorporating the homemade face masks, herbal infusions, or traditional massage techniques we have discussed into your skincare regimen.

Furthermore, don't be afraid to explore the wisdom of your ancestors by seeking guidance from knowledgeable practitioners or elders within your community. They can provide valuable insights and share their expertise on how to incorporate these remedies into your daily life in a meaningful and sustainable way.

By embracing these ancestral remedies and incorporating them into your daily routines, you can establish a self-care practice that honors your heritage while nurturing your mind, body, and spirit. Remember, self-care is a journey, and by infusing it with the wisdom of the past, you can create a sustainable practice that supports your overall well-being.

Developing Rituals and Habits for Long-Term Well-Being

I recently attended a conference where the importance of having a seat belt in life was emphasized to me. It serves as a kind of restrictive stability, acting as a safety net in our ever-changing world.

Living in today's times, it is crucial to prioritize our well-being. One effective way to do this is by developing rituals and habits that support long-term holistic well-being. These rituals and habits act as anchors in our lives, providing stability, balance, and a sense of purpose. They help us navigate the challenges and uncertainties that life throws our way, ensuring that we maintain our physical, mental, and emotional well-being.

Rituals and habits have a profound impact on our overall well-being. They create a sense of structure and routine, which can be particularly beneficial during times of stress or transition. By engaging in consistent practices, we cultivate a sense of discipline and self-care, allowing us to better manage our energy and focus. Whether it's starting the day with a mindfulness meditation, practicing gratitude before bed, or engaging in regular exercise, these rituals and habits become the building blocks of a healthy and fulfilling life.

When developing rituals and habits for long-term well-being, it is important to consider the holistic nature of our well-being. For example, incorporating activities such as journaling, spending time in nature, or engaging in creative pursuits can nurture our emotional and spiritual selves. Similarly, prioritizing sleep, maintaining a balanced diet, and engaging in regular physical activity contribute to our physical well-being.

Consistency is key when it comes to developing rituals and habits. It is important to commit to these practices and integrate them into our daily lives. Start small and gradually build upon them, allowing them to become second nature. Surround yourself with a supportive environment that encourages and reinforces these habits. Whether it's finding an accountability partner, joining a community of like-minded individuals, or utilizing technology to track your progress, these external factors can greatly enhance your success in developing and maintaining these rituals and habits.

By incorporating consistent practices into our daily lives, we create a solid foundation for our physical, mental, and emotional well-being. These rituals and habits act as anchors, providing stability and balance amidst the challenges of life.

Consistency and discipline play a crucial role in integrating ancestral remedies into daily life. By adhering to these principles, we can effectively incorporate these remedies into our existing routines and create new habits that promote overall health and vitality.

Discipline plays a crucial role in cultivating a lifestyle of holistic health. It is the key that unlocks the door to long-term well-being and overall balance. When we talk about holistic health, we refer to the integration of physical, mental, and emotional well-being. It is about nurturing all aspects of our being to achieve optimal health and harmony.

Discipline provides the structure and consistency needed to make positive choices and maintain healthy habits. It empowers us to prioritize self-care, such as regular exercise, nutritious eating, and sufficient rest. By adhering to a disciplined routine, we create a solid foundation for our physical health, allowing our bodies to function optimally and ward off illness.

Moreover, discipline extends beyond physical health. It encompasses mental and emotional well-being as well. Through discipline, we can cultivate mindfulness practices, such as meditation or journaling, which help us manage stress, enhance focus, and promote emotional resilience. It encourages us to engage in activities that nourish our minds, such as reading, learning, and pursuing creative outlets.

Discipline also plays a vital role in breaking unhealthy patterns and overcoming addictions. It requires commitment, self-control, and the willingness to make difficult choices. By practicing discipline, we can replace destructive habits with positive ones, leading to a more balanced and fulfilling life.

Discipline is the cornerstone of a holistic approach to health. It empowers us to make conscious choices, establish healthy habits, and maintain balance in all aspects of our lives. By embracing discipline, we can unlock our full potential and cultivate a lifestyle of holistic well-being.

Here are some practical tips and strategies to achieve this integration:

- Start with a Clear Intention: Begin by setting a clear intention to incorporate ancestral remedies into your daily life. This intention will serve as a guiding force and help you stay focused on your goals.

- Educate Yourself: Take the time to educate yourself about the specific ancestral remedies you wish to incorporate. Learn about their benefits, usage, and any precautions or contraindications. This knowledge will empower you to make informed decisions and use the remedies effectively.

- Create a Routine: Establish a consistent routine for incorporating ancestral remedies. This could involve designating specific times of the day for their use, such as morning or evening rituals. Consistency is key to making these remedies a regular part of your life.

- Start Small: Begin by incorporating one ancestral remedy at a time. Trying to incorporate too many remedies at once can be overwhelming and unsustainable. Start with one remedy that resonates with you and gradually add others as you become comfortable.

- Set Reminders: Use reminders, such as alarms or sticky notes, to prompt you to take your ancestral remedies. This will help you stay on track and ensure that you don't forget to incorporate them into your daily routine.

- Adapt to Your Existing Routine: Look for opportunities to seamlessly integrate ancestral remedies into your existing routines. For example, if you already have a morning skincare routine, consider adding a herbal face mask or incorporating herbal teas into your breakfast routine.

- Seek Support: Connect with like-minded individuals who are also interested in ancestral remedies. Join online communities, attend workshops, or find a mentor who can provide guidance and support on your journey. Sharing experiences and learning from others can be motivating and inspiring.

- Track Your Progress: Keep a journal or use a tracking app to monitor your progress. Note any changes you observe in your overall health and well-being. This will serve as a reminder of the positive impact ancestral remedies are having on your life.

- Be Patient and Persistent: Integrating ancestral remedies into your daily life is a process that requires patience and persistence. Results may not be immediate, but with consistent practice, you will begin to experience the benefits over time.

- Celebrate Milestones: Celebrate your milestones and achievements along the way. Recognize and acknowledge the efforts you are putting into incorporating ancestral remedies into your daily life. This will help you stay motivated and committed to your journey.

By embracing consistency and discipline, and following these practical tips and strategies, you can successfully integrate ancestral remedies into your daily life. Embracing these remedies will not only promote overall health and vitality but also connect you to the wisdom of your ancestors.

Overcoming Challenges and Obstacles in Implementing Ancestral Remedies

Overcoming challenges and obstacles in implementing ancestral remedies involves utilizing practical solutions and tools to stay motivated and committed throughout the process. These challenges may arise from societal skepticism or lack of awareness about the effectiveness of ancestral remedies. Additionally, personal barriers, such as self-doubt or limited resources, can hinder progress.

However, by staying determined and seeking support from like-minded individuals or communities, one can overcome these obstacles. It is crucial to educate other women about the benefits of ancestral remedies and share success stories to inspire and encourage others to embrace these traditional healing practices. By doing so, we can preserve and promote the wisdom of our ancestors while improving our overall well-being.

Navigating Resistance from External Sources

- Educating Family and Friends: Communicate the benefits and importance of ancestral remedies to your loved ones, addressing any misconceptions or skepticism they may have.

- Seeking Community Support: Join local or online communities that share your interest in ancestral remedies. Connect with like-minded individuals who can provide encouragement and advice.

- Engaging with Experts: Consult with practitioners or experts in ancestral remedies who can guide you through the process and help you address any external resistance you may encounter.

Overcoming Personal Barriers

- Self-Education: Invest time in learning about the science, history, and cultural significance of ancestral remedies. This knowledge will strengthen your belief in their efficacy and help you overcome personal doubts.

- Setting Realistic Goals: Start small and gradually incorporate ancestral remedies into your daily routine. Setting achievable goals will prevent overwhelm and increase your chances of long-term success.

- Building Consistency: Establish a consistent practice by incorporating ancestral remedies into your daily rituals. Create a schedule or set reminders to ensure you stay committed to the integration process.

- Tracking Progress: Keep a journal or record of your experiences with ancestral remedies. Document any positive changes or benefits you observe, which will serve as motivation during challenging times.

- Self-Care and Mindfulness: Prioritize self-care practices that support your overall well-being. Engage in activities such as meditation, yoga, or journaling to cultivate a positive mindset and maintain motivation.

Practical Solutions and Tools

- Adapting Ancestral Remedies to Modern Life: Explore ways to integrate ancestral remedies into your current lifestyle. This may involve adapting traditional practices to fit your daily routine or finding alternative methods that align with your preferences.

- Creating Rituals: Develop personalized rituals that incorporate ancestral remedies. Rituals can provide structure, meaning, and a sense of connection to your heritage, making the integration process more fulfilling.

- Seeking Professional Guidance: Consult with holistic health practitioners or herbalists who specialize in ancestral remedies. They can provide personalized guidance, recommend specific remedies, and help you navigate any challenges you may face.

- Utilizing Technology: Leverage technology to enhance your integration journey. Use mobile apps, online resources, or virtual platforms to access information, connect with experts, and track your progress.

Incorporating ancestral remedies into daily routines can unlock numerous benefits for physical, mental, and emotional health. Creating a self-care plan that integrates ancestral remedies requires identifying specific remedies that align with individual needs and goals. Understanding heritage and cultural background helps tap into a rich source of knowledge and wisdom for creating a self-care plan that is aligned with our roots.

Exploring ancestral healing remedies involves researching, consulting knowledgeable individuals, and experimenting with different remedies to find what works best.

As we've seen, practical aspects of incorporating ancestral remedies include sourcing natural ingredients, learning how to prepare remedies, and creating a sustainable practice.

Developing rituals and habits that support long-term well-being is crucial for maintaining stability, balance, and a sense of purpose. Consistency, discipline, and commitment are key in integrating ancestral remedies into daily life.

Finally, overcoming challenges and obstacles in implementing ancestral remedies requires navigating external resistance and personal barriers, as well as utilizing practical solutions and tools to stay motivated and committed. None of this is easy work, but it is so worthwhile. You've come so far already.

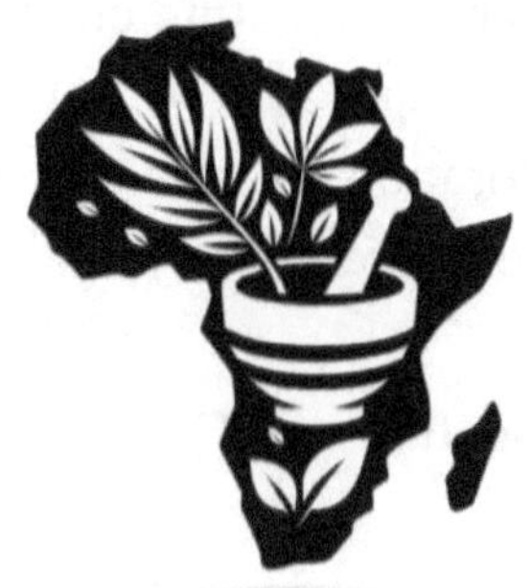

Chapter 9
Cultural Heritage and Self-Care

Congratulations once more for making it this far. In Chapter 9, we will delve into the profound significance of cultural heritage as a foundation for self-care. We will explore how honoring and preserving our cultural identity can contribute to our overall well-being. Cultural heritage encompasses the customs, traditions, beliefs, and values passed down through generations, shaping our sense of self and providing a rich tapestry of practices that can enhance our self-care routines.

In this chapter, we will delve deeper into the connection between cultural identity and self-care practices. We will explore how embracing and celebrating our cultural heritage can empower us to nurture our physical, mental, and emotional well-being. By acknowledging and valuing our cultural roots, we can tap into a wealth of wisdom and rituals that have stood the test of time.

Furthermore, this chapter will shed light on the diverse rituals and practices specific to different cultural backgrounds. From ancient healing techniques to unexplored *mindfulness practices, we will uncover a treasure trove of self-care rituals that have been passed down through generations. By incorporating these practices into our daily routines, we can cultivate a deeper connection with ourselves and our cultural heritage.

Embracing our roots and integrating cultural practices can lead to a more holistic and fulfilling approach to well-being. Let us continue on this transformative exploration together, as we unlock the power of cultural heritage in our self-care journey.

Understanding the Importance of Cultural Identity in Self-Care Practices

Cultural identity plays a vital role in shaping a woman's self-care practices and her overall well-being. Exploring and understanding one's cultural identity can help develop a deeper connection to one's roots and enhance their self-care routines.

In this section, we will look at the ways in which cultural identity influences self-care choices and the benefits of aligning self-care practices with one's cultural heritage.

Understanding the importance of cultural identity in self-care practices is crucial for promoting holistic well-being. Cultural identity encompasses the beliefs, values, traditions, and customs that shape an individual's sense of self and their connection to their community. When it comes to self-care, acknowledging and embracing one's cultural identity can have profound effects on mental, emotional, and physical health.

Firstly, cultural identity provides a sense of belonging and rootedness, which is essential for self-care. Engaging in practices that are deeply rooted in one's culture can foster a sense of comfort, familiarity, and security. For example, participating in traditional rituals, such as meditation or prayer, can promote relaxation and inner peace. These practices not only nourish the individual but also strengthen their connection to their cultural heritage.

Secondly, cultural identity influences the perception of well-being and self-care. Different cultures have unique perspectives on what constitutes a healthy lifestyle. For instance, some cultures prioritize communal activities and social connections as integral components of self-care. In contrast, others may emphasize solitude and introspection. Understanding these cultural nuances allows individuals to tailor their self-care practices to align with their cultural values, resulting in a more meaningful and effective self-care routine.

Moreover, cultural identity shapes the availability and accessibility of self-care resources. Cultural communities often have their own traditional healing practices, herbal remedies, and wellness techniques that have been passed down through generations. Incorporating these culturally specific resources into self-care routines can provide individuals with a sense of empowerment and connection to their heritage.

By embracing and honoring cultural traditions, women can cultivate a deeper sense of self, find solace in their cultural heritage, and access resources that are uniquely tailored to their needs. Understanding the interplay between cultural identity and self-care allows us to embark on a journey of self-discovery and self-nurturing that is both meaningful and transformative.

Cultural identity plays a significant role in shaping who we are as individuals. By delving into our cultural heritage and traditions, we gain insights into the rich history and experiences of our ancestors. This knowledge allows us to appreciate the struggles, triumphs, and contributions of those who came before us. It enables us to develop a greater appreciation for our cultural heritage and instills a sense of pride in our identity.

Furthermore, exploring cultural identity can contribute to personal growth and self-discovery. As we learn more about our cultural background, we become more aware of our own values, beliefs, and customs. This self-awareness helps us understand why we think and act the way we do. It allows us to embrace our uniqueness and develop a more authentic and meaningful sense of self. By understanding our cultural identity, we gain insights into the experiences that have shaped us and can use this knowledge to navigate life's challenges with greater confidence and resilience.

Moreover, exploring cultural identity can enhance our self-care routines. Cultural practices often incorporate rituals and traditions that promote well-being and balance. Whether it's through meditation, dance, cuisine, or other cultural activities, engaging with our cultural heritage can provide a sense of comfort, connection, and purpose. These practices can serve as mindful reminders to prioritize self-care, leading to improved mental, emotional, and physical health.

Exploring our roots can enrich our lives in numerous ways. We can develop a deeper appreciation for who we are and create a strong foundation for a fulfilling and meaningful life.

Cultural identity plays a significant role in shaping self-care choices. Cultural self-care practices often incorporate holistic approaches that address physical, mental, and spiritual well-being. This comprehensive approach promotes overall wellness and balance. Additionally, cultural self-care practices can offer a unique perspective on self-care, re-introducing women to diverse healing modalities and alternative therapies.

By honoring our cultural heritage, we can enhance our self-care journey and cultivate a deeper understanding of ourselves.

Exploring rituals and practices specific to different cultural backgrounds

Cultural diversity is a beautiful aspect of our world, and within each culture, there are unique rituals and practices that contribute to self-care and well-being. These rituals and practices are often deeply rooted in traditions, customs, and beliefs that have been passed down through generations. They serve as a source of connection, meaning, and solace for individuals within their respective cultural backgrounds. In this section, we will explore various cultural backgrounds and highlight specific rituals and practices that promote self-care.

Asian Cultures

Meditation and Mindfulness: Asian cultures, such as Buddhism and Zen, have long embraced meditation and mindfulness practices as means of achieving inner peace, clarity, and balance. Techniques such as breath awareness, sitting meditation, and mindful walking are widely employed in Buddhist practices to foster a serene and mindful state of mind. These techniques, rooted in ancient wisdom, offer profound insights into the nature of the mind and provide practical tools for personal growth and self-discovery.

Breath awareness is a fundamental technique in Buddhist meditation. It involves directing one's attention to the breath, observing its natural rhythm and flow. By focusing on the breath, practitioners develop a heightened sense of present-moment awareness, anchoring themselves in the here and now. This technique cultivates a deep sense of calm and tranquility, allowing individuals to let go of distractions and connect with their inner selves.

Sitting meditation, also known as zazen, is another powerful technique in Buddhist practice. It involves finding a comfortable posture and bringing attention to the present moment. During sitting meditation, practitioners observe their thoughts and emotions without judgment, allowing them to arise and pass away naturally. This practice cultivates mindfulness and equanimity, enabling individuals to develop a deeper understanding of the impermanent and ever-changing nature of existence.

Mindful walking is a technique that combines meditation with physical movement. It involves walking slowly and deliberately, paying close attention to each step and the sensations in the body. Mindful walking encourages practitioners to be fully present in the act of walking, bringing awareness to the sensations of the feet touching the ground, the movement of the body, and the surrounding environment. This practice enhances mindfulness in everyday activities, fostering a sense of interconnectedness with the world around us.**

These Buddhist techniques go beyond mere relaxation exercises; they are profound tools for self-transformation and spiritual development.

Through consistent practice, we can cultivate a deep sense of inner peace, clarity, and compassion. These are hallmarks of holistic wellness. These techniques not only benefit the individual but also have the potential to positively impact relationships, work, and overall well-being.

Tea Ceremonies: Tea ceremonies, prevalent in cultures like Japan and China, are elevated rituals where the preparation and consumption of tea become an act of mindfulness and meditation. These ceremonies offer a serene escape from the chaos of everyday life, fostering a deep connection with nature and allowing participants to savor the beauty of simplicity in everyday life. Through the harmonious blend of precise movements, serene surroundings, and the delicate aroma of tea, tea ceremonies create a space for tranquility, reflection, and an appreciation for life's small joys. Gratitude and holistic health are widely known to go hand in hand.

Native American Cultures

Sweat Lodges: Sweats lodges, commonly used by Native American tribes, are ceremonial structures where people engage in intense heat and steam sessions. These rituals are seen as a way to purify the body, mind, and spirit, and promote physical and spiritual healing. They serve as spaces for individuals to partake in intense heat and steam sessions. These rituals hold significant cultural and spiritual importance, as they are believed to cleanse and purify the body, mind, and spirit. Moreover, sweat lodges are considered to facilitate physical and spiritual healing processes.

Smudging: Many Native American cultures practice smudging, a purification ritual that involves burning sacred herbs, such as sage or sweetgrass, to cleanse the energy of a space or individual. Smudging is believed to release negative or stagnant energies and restore balance and harmony.

African Cultures

Dance and Drumming: Dance and drumming have deep cultural significance in many African countries. These expressive forms of movement and rhythm are not only sources of joy and celebration but also serve as means of self-expression, connection with ancestral traditions, and physical well-being.

In African communities, creativity and joy are recognized as essential components of holistic health. The act of engaging in creative activities, such as dance and drumming, allows individuals to tap into their inner creativity, express themselves authentically, and experience a sense of liberation. This not only enhances mental and emotional health but also contributes to physical fitness and vitality.

The rhythmic movements and energetic beats of dance and drumming stimulate the body, promoting cardiovascular health, coordination, and strength. Moreover, these cultural practices foster a sense of community and connection, as they are often performed collectively, bringing people together in a shared experience of joy and unity.These practices continue to be cherished and celebrated as vital aspects of well-being, both within African communities and the diaspora.

Ancestral Worship: Ancestral worship is prevalent in various African cultures, where individuals pay reverence to their ancestors through rituals and ceremonies. These practices provide a sense of connection to one's roots, wisdom from previous generations, and a feeling of guidance and protection. Ancestral worship is an integral part of the * concept of Sankofa, which emphasizes the importance of honoring and learning from our past as we navigate our present and shape our future.

Indigenous Cultures

Nature Connection: Indigenous cultures around the world emphasize the importance of connecting with nature as a means of self-care. Spending time in natural environments, engaging in activities like forest bathing, and recognizing the interconnectedness of all living beings are practices that promote spiritual well-being and a sense of harmony.

^^Here's a short practice example for anyone who might wish to try:

Find a peaceful forest or wooded area near you. Take a slow, leisurely walk, paying close attention to your surroundings. Notice the sounds of birds chirping, the rustling of leaves, and the scent of the forest. As you walk, allow yourself to fully immerse in the present moment, letting go of any worries or distractions. Take deep breaths, inhaling the fresh air and exhaling any tension or stress. Feel the connection between yourself and the natural world around you. Take your time and enjoy the rejuvenating experience of a guided forest bath.

Vision Quests: Vision quests are ancient practices that have been carried out by many Indigenous communities for centuries. They involve embarking on a profound and transformative journey of self-discovery, personal guidance, and spiritual growth. During a vision quest, individuals immerse themselves in solitude and fasting while being surrounded by the beauty and serenity of nature.

The purpose of a vision quest is to seek deep insights, clarity, and connection to the universe. It is believed that by disconnecting from the distractions of everyday life and immersing oneself in the natural world, one can tap into their inner wisdom and receive guidance from the spiritual realm.

The process of a vision quest typically involves finding a secluded and sacred location in nature, such as a mountain, forest, or desert. The individual then spends a significant period of time alone, often ranging from a few days to several weeks, depending on the specific tradition and purpose of the quest.

During this time of solitude, fasting, and contemplation, participants engage in various practices such as meditation, prayer, reflection, and sometimes even physical challenges. These practices are designed to quiet the mind, open the heart, and create a receptive state for receiving visions, messages, and insights.

The visions and experiences that occur during a vision quest are highly personal and unique to each individual. They can manifest in the form of vivid dreams, symbolic encounters with animals or natural elements, or profound moments of clarity and revelation. These experiences are often seen as messages from the spiritual realm, guiding the individual towards their purpose, path, and personal growth.

Upon completion of the vision quest, individuals return to their community with a renewed sense of self, a deeper understanding of their place in the world, and a heightened connection to the spiritual and natural realms. The insights gained during the quest can be integrated into their daily lives, guiding their decisions, actions, and relationships.

It is important to note that vision quests are deeply rooted in Indigenous cultures and hold significant spiritual and cultural significance. They are not to be taken lightly or approached as a mere recreational activity. Respect for the traditions, protocols, and teachings associated with vision quests is essential when engaging with this practice.

Overall, vision quests offer a profound opportunity for individuals to embark on a transformative journey of self-discovery, personal growth, and spiritual connection. They provide a sacred space for seeking guidance, gaining insights, and deepening one's relationship with oneself and the universe.

Middle Eastern Cultures

Hammams: Hammams, or Turkish baths, are traditional bathing and cleansing rituals that have been practiced in Middle Eastern cultures for centuries. These communal spaces provide a sanctuary for relaxation, rejuvenation, and purification of the body and mind.

Islamic Prayer: Islamic prayer, performed five times a day, is not only a religious obligation but also a means of self-care and connection with a higher power. The act of prayer allows individuals to pause, reflect, and find inner peace amidst the busyness of daily life.

Exploring rituals and practices specific to different cultural backgrounds can broaden our perspectives and deepen our understanding of self-care. Each culture has its own unique traditions and customs that promote well-being and provide comfort and solace to individuals within their communities. By embracing and respecting these practices, we can learn valuable lessons about self-care, mindfulness, and the interconnectedness of humanity as a whole.

Learning how to honor and preserve cultural heritage through self-care

Self-care is not just about taking care of our physical, mental, and emotional well-being; it can also serve as a powerful tool for honoring and preserving our cultural heritage. By incorporating elements of our cultural traditions, rituals, and practices into our self-care routines, we can deepen our connection to our roots and ensure that our cultural heritage thrives for generations to come.

As we have seen, one way to honor and preserve cultural heritage through self-care is by embracing and practicing traditional healing methods. By incorporating these traditional healing methods into our self-care routine, we not only promote our own well-being but also keep alive the knowledge and wisdom of our ancestors.

Another way to honor and preserve cultural heritage through self-care is by celebrating and participating in cultural festivals and events. These events provide opportunities to engage with our cultural traditions, music, dance, and cuisine. By actively participating in these celebrations, we not only create beautiful memories but also contribute to the preservation of our cultural heritage. We can also support local artisans and craftsmen who create traditional handicrafts and products, allowing us to showcase and maintain the unique artistry and craftsmanship of our culture.

Moreover, learning about our cultural history, storytelling, and passing down traditions to future generations can be a form of self-care and a way to honor and preserve our cultural heritage. By taking the time to research and understand the significance of cultural practices, we can gain a deeper appreciation for our heritage and make a conscious effort to continue these traditions within our families and communities.

Self-care activities that involve cultural exploration, such as reading literature from our culture, learning traditional dances, or cooking traditional recipes, can also be meaningful ways to honor and preserve our cultural heritage. These activities not only provide personal enjoyment and fulfillment but also create a bridge between generations and foster a sense of pride and continuity.

By incorporating elements of our culture into our self-care routines and passing down traditions, we ensure that our cultural heritage remains alive and vibrant. Self-care not only benefits us individually but also contributes to the preservation of our identity and the rich tapestry of human diversity. Let's take a look at this last part.

Cultural traditions and practices are the threads that weave together the rich tapestry of our heritage. They are the essence of who we are, connecting us to our roots and shaping our identity. In a rapidly changing world, it is crucial to recognize the significance of passing down these traditions to future generations. One powerful way to achieve this is through the practice of self-care.

Self-care, though often associated with personal well-being, goes beyond individual benefits. It can serve as a vessel for preserving and transmitting cultural traditions. By engaging in self-care practices rooted in our cultural heritage, we not only nurture our own physical and mental health but also ensure the continuity of our traditions.

When we prioritize self-care, we create opportunities to immerse ourselves in cultural practices that have been passed down for generations. Whether it's practicing meditation, preparing traditional meals, or participating in rituals, these activities become more than just self-care, they become acts of cultural preservation.

Passing down cultural traditions through self-care is a way to honor our ancestors and keep their legacy alive. It allows us to connect with our roots, fostering a sense of belonging and pride in our cultural heritage. Moreover, it provides a platform for intergenerational exchange, where elders can share their wisdom and younger generations can learn and appreciate their cultural heritage.

In the final chapter of this book, we will look at how women can be empowered overall through our ancestral wisdom.

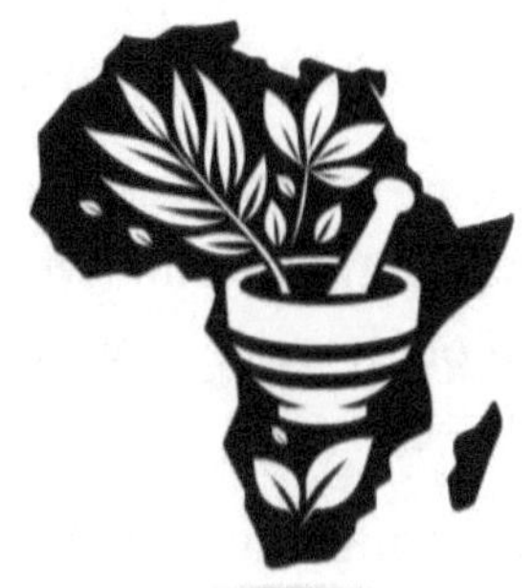

Chapter 10
Empowering Women Through Ancestral Wisdom

In this final chapter of our guidebook, we will delve into a topic close to my heart—empowering women to take control of their health and well-being through the use of ancestral wisdom.

Throughout herstory, women have been the keepers of ancient knowledge, passed down through maternal lineages. It is time for us to embrace this wisdom and harness its power.

Within these final pages, we will explore the significance of women embracing their ancestral wisdom. Holistic self-care practices have transformative effects as a form of empowerment. By prioritizing our own well-being, we can better serve ourselves and those around us.

Moreover, this chapter provides a wealth of tools and resources for continued growth and self-discovery. From practical tips to ancient rituals, I aim to equip women with the knowledge and support they need to thrive in all aspects of their lives.

It is my intention that you enjoy this empowering journey as we tap into the wisdom of our ancestors and unlock the true potential that lies within each and every one of us.

Embracing Your Divine Feminine Ancestral Wisdom

Embracing our ancestral wisdom as women is a transformative journey that can profoundly impact our lives. By connecting with the wisdom and knowledge of our ancestors, we can tap into a rich source of power, strength, and resilience.

Understanding and honoring the knowledge and practices passed down through generations of women, especially Black women, is of utmost importance. It allows us to recognize our heritage and lineage, providing us with a sense of belonging and connection to something greater than ourselves. We don't often get this much ownership of our spiritual, mental, emotional, and physical lives. This connection acts as a grounding force, offering support during uncertain times and adversity.

Ancestral wisdom offers women a wealth of knowledge and practices that have stood the test of time. From herbal remedies for health and healing to rituals for self-care and self-expression, these practices are rooted in deep wisdom and intuition. Additionally, the stories and folklore passed down provide valuable life lessons, making ancestral wisdom a treasure trove of practical and profound teachings.

Embracing ancestral wisdom means embracing one's unique heritage and cultural identity. Each woman carries within her a tapestry of cultural traditions and customs, shaping their identity. Exploring and celebrating these roots not only deepens self-understanding but also contributes to the preservation and enrichment of their heritage.

Moreover, embracing ancestral wisdom empowers women to reclaim their voice and agency. It enables them to challenge societal norms and expectations that may restrict their potential. By drawing on the wisdom and strength of their ancestors, women can find the courage to break free from patriarchal structures and embrace their authentic selves.

By embracing our heritage and cultural identity, women not only transform their own lives but also leave a positive impact on future generations.

Self-Care as a form of Empowerment

Self-care is not just about pampering oneself or indulging in temporary pleasures. It is an essential practice that empowers women to prioritize their well-being and reclaim control over their lives. By engaging in intentional self-care practices, women can cultivate a strong sense of empowerment and create a foundation of self-love and resilience.

At its core, self-care involves nurturing and nourishing oneself in all aspects - physically, mentally, emotionally, and spiritually. It means setting boundaries, saying no to things that deplete energy, and saying yes to activities that bring joy and fulfillment. It is about tuning in to your own needs and desires, and giving yourself permission to prioritize them.

Self-care as a form of empowerment goes beyond the superficial. It is about reclaiming ownership of your body, mind, and emotions. It is about recognizing that taking care of yourself is not selfish but necessary for overall well-being. When women prioritize self-care, we send a powerful message that our needs and happiness matter.

Inspiring self-care practices can encompass a wide range of activities, depending on individual preferences and needs. It may involve engaging in regular exercise, practicing mindfulness and meditation, nourishing the body with nutritious food, getting enough rest and sleep, engaging in creative expression, spending time in nature, seeking therapy or counseling, or simply indulging in activities that bring joy and relaxation.

By embracing self-care as a form of empowerment, women can cultivate a deep sense of self-worth, resilience, and inner strength. It enables us to show up fully in our personal and professional lives, set healthy boundaries, and make choices that align with our values and aspirations. Ultimately, inspiring self-care practices not only benefit individual women but also contribute to creating a culture that values and supports women's well-being and empowerment.

Prioritizing self-care is crucial for overall well-being. It allows women to recharge, reduce stress, and improve mental and physical health. By making self-care a priority, we can experience increased happiness, resilience, and the ability to navigate challenges with greater ease.

It's important to reconnect with ancestral wisdom and embrace practices that nourish our mind, body, and soul. Engaging in rituals, such as lighting candles or burning incense, can help create a sense of calm and grounding. Meditation allows us to quiet our minds and find inner peace. And spending time in nature, whether it's a walk in the park or tending to a garden, helps us reconnect with the natural world and rejuvenate our spirits. By remembering to incorporate these self-care practices into our daily lives, we can cultivate a deeper sense of balance and harmony.

Tools and Resources for Continued Growth and Self-Discovery

This subpoint will provide practical tools and resources that women can utilize to further their personal growth and self-discovery journey.

It will discuss books, websites, workshops, and other sources of information that can support women in exploring and expanding their understanding of ancestral wisdom.

Tips for integrating these tools and resources into daily life will be provided.

"'Providing tools and resources for continued growth and self-discovery'"

In the following section, I will equip you with practical tools and resources that can support your ongoing personal growth and self-discovery journey. By exploring]g accessible and effective resources, women can be empowered to tap into their potential, develop new skills, and deepen their understanding of themselves. Here are some key tools and resources that can aid in this process:

Personal Development Books: Books are a valuable source of knowledge and inspiration. Recommending books on personal development, self-help, and psychology can provide women with insights, strategies, and practical advice to navigate their personal growth journey. Here are some popular titles:

1. "Becoming" by Michelle Obama: This empowering memoir by Michelle Obama shares her journey from the South Side of Chicago to the White House. It offers insights into personal growth, resilience, and the power of determination.

2. "The Power of Now" by Eckhart Tolle: This book explores the concept of living in the present moment and finding inner peace. It offers guidance on how to let go of past regrets and future anxieties, and embrace where you are now.

3. "Daring Greatly" by Brené Brown: In this book, Brené Brown explores the importance of vulnerability and embracing imperfections. She encourages readers to step out of their comfort zones, be authentic, and cultivate meaningful connections.

4. "Mindset" by Carol S. Dweck: This book delves into the concept of mindset and how it affects our success and personal growth. It explores the difference between a fixed mindset and a growth mindset, and provides strategies to develop a growth mindset for achieving goals.

These books offer valuable insights, practical tools, and inspiration for personal development. Happy reading!

Online Courses and Workshops: The internet offers a vast array of online courses and workshops covering various topics related to personal growth and self-discovery. These courses provide structured learning experiences and allow women to explore specific areas of interest at their own pace. Platforms like Coursera, Udemy, and Skillshare offer a wide range of courses on topics such as mindfulness, emotional intelligence, goal setting, and communication skills.

Journaling Prompts: Journaling is a powerful tool for self-reflection and self-discovery. Prompts can be focused on gratitude, personal values, life goals, or exploring limiting beliefs. By regularly engaging in journaling, women can gain clarity, process their experiences, and uncover new insights about themselves.

Here are some journaling prompts specifically designed for women to explore their thoughts, emotions, and aspirations:

- Reflect on a time when you felt the most empowered. What were the circumstances, and how did it make you feel?

- Write about a woman who inspires you and why. What qualities or achievements do you admire in her?

- Describe a challenge or obstacle you have overcome in your life. How did you navigate through it, and what did you learn from the experience?

- What are your top three values in life? How do these values shape your decisions and actions?

- Imagine your ideal future self. What does she look like, and what accomplishments has she achieved? How can you work towards becoming her?

- Write a letter to your younger self. What advice or words of encouragement would you give her?

- What are your biggest dreams and aspirations? How can you break them down into smaller, actionable steps?

- Explore your relationship with self-care. What activities or practices make you feel nourished, rejuvenated, and connected to yourself?

- Write about a time when you took a risk and stepped out of your comfort zone. How did it impact your personal growth?

- Reflect on a recent success or achievement. What strengths and skills did you utilize to accomplish it?

Remember, journaling is a personal and introspective practice. Feel free to adapt these prompts to suit your individual needs and interests. Happy journaling!

Meditation and Mindfulness Apps: Mindfulness and meditation practices can enhance self-awareness, reduce stress, and promote overall well-being. Popular meditation and mindfulness apps like Headspace, Calm, or Insight Timer can give women access to guided meditations, breathing exercises, and mindfulness practices that can be incorporated into their daily routines.

Supportive Communities: Connecting with like-minded individuals who are also on a personal growth journey can be incredibly beneficial. I encourage women to join supportive communities, whether online or in-person, which can provide a sense of belonging, accountability, and opportunities for shared learning. Platforms like Meetup, Facebook groups, or local community centers often host events and gatherings focused on personal growth and self-discovery.

Coaching and Mentoring: Engaging with a professional coach or mentor can provide personalized guidance and support in navigating personal growth and self-discovery. Coaches and mentors can help you set goals, overcome challenges, and develop strategies for personal development. Researching and recommending reputable coaching services or mentorship programs can be invaluable for women seeking individualized support.

By providing these tools and resources through my books, I aim to empower women to continue their journey of personal growth and self-discovery. Remember, each person's journey is unique, and it's important to explore different resources and find what resonates best with individual needs and preferences.

Exploring Ancestral Wisdom: Tools and Resources for Women

In the journey of self-discovery and personal growth, exploring ancestral wisdom can be a profound and transformative experience. For women seeking to connect with their roots and expand their understanding of ancestral wisdom, there are various tools and resources available. This section will delve into books, websites, workshops, and other sources of information that can support women in their exploration. Additionally, practical tips for integrating these tools and resources into daily life will be provided.

Books: Books serve as gateways to knowledge and wisdom, offering insights into different cultures, traditions, and ancestral practices. There are numerous books that focus on ancestral wisdom, providing guidance on topics such as herbal medicine, rituals, folklore, and spirituality. Some notable titles include "Women Who Run with the Wolves" by Clarissa Pinkola Estés, "The Spiral Dance" by Starhawk, and "The Book of Symbols" by Taschen. My favorite book to recommend is S'Otito by Yoruba priestess Ola Omi Amalokunde. Her blurb states:

Within these pages is the understanding that our Ancestors carried of how life is created, sustained & maintained from generation to generation. Gathered through 20 years of study of West Afrikan culture & spirituality these truths are revealed to you in 18 simply written lesson

By immersing yourself in these literary treasures, you can gain a deeper understanding of your ancestral heritage.

Websites: The digital age has made information more accessible than ever before. Websites dedicated to ancestral wisdom offer a wealth of resources, articles, and forums for women to explore. Websites like Ancestral Wisdom, Ancient Origins, and Sacred Earth provide a platform for sharing knowledge, connecting with like-minded individuals, and accessing a vast array of information on ancestral practices. These online communities can be invaluable in supporting women on their journey of exploration.

Workshops and Retreats: Attending workshops and retreats focused on ancestral wisdom can be a transformative experience. These immersive environments provide opportunities to learn from experienced practitioners, engage in hands-on activities, and connect with a community of individuals who share a similar interest. Workshops may cover topics such as ancestral healing, shamanic practices, or indigenous wisdom. Retreats offer a chance to disconnect from the demands of daily life and fully immerse oneself in the exploration of ancestral traditions.

Other Sources of Information

In addition to books, websites, and workshops, there are other sources of information that can support women in their quest for ancestral wisdom. Podcasts, documentaries, and online courses provide alternative avenues for learning and exploration. Listening to podcasts like "The Ancestral Healing Podcast" or watching documentaries like "The Wisdom of the Grandmothers" can offer valuable insights and inspiration. Online courses, such as those offered by organizations like The Shift Network or Udemy, provide structured learning experiences that can be tailored to individual interests and schedules.

Tips for Integration

To make the most of these tools and resources, it is important to integrate them into daily life. Here are some practical tips:

- Create a dedicated space: Set up a sacred space in your home where you can engage in ancestral practices, read books, or listen to podcasts.

- Establish a routine: Set aside regular time each day or week to engage with ancestral wisdom. This could be through reading, participating in online courses, or practicing rituals.

- Connect with others: Join online communities or local groups where you can share experiences, ask questions, and learn from others on a similar path.

- Embrace ancestral practices: Incorporate ancestral rituals, such as creating altars, working with herbs, or practicing meditation, into your daily life.

By utilizing books, websites, workshops, and other sources of information, women can embark on a journey of exploring and expanding their understanding of ancestral wisdom and holistic well-being. Integrating these tools and resources into daily life can deepen connection with ancestral heritage and foster personal growth. Embrace the richness of ancestral wisdom and let it guide you on a transformative path of self-discovery.

Conclusion and Book Key Takeaways

Congratulations for making it to the end of this guidebook.

We have done a lot of work at this point, having explored various cultural practices and traditions that can enhance holistic wellness and contribute to self-transformation and spiritual development. We've covered practices rooted in different cultural backgrounds, such as African, African American, Buddhist, Native American, Middle Eastern, and Indigenous cultures.

I hope I have emphasized the importance of honoring and preserving cultural heritage through self-care, along with the significance of passing down cultural traditions and practices.

Through this offering, you now have with you handy tools and practical tips for integrating these practices into daily life. You can always go back to your list of plants, herbs, rituals, and ceremonies to incorporate for balanced well-being and holistic women's health.

The wisdom and resilience of Black women in healthcare shows the connection between the Divine Feminine and addressing the necessity of holistic health. Embracing holistic approaches and ancestral cures promotes well-being, transformation, and self-empowerment. We have seen this in the examples of the deep connection Indigenous cultures have with nature-based practices and the benefits of honoring and celebrating cultural heritage in self-care routines.

You have begun a life-changing journey, and the real fun of regular integration in your daily life as a powerful woman begins now.

Key Takeaways:

- Cultural practices and traditions from various backgrounds can enhance holistic wellness and self-transformation.

- Self-care should include honoring and preserving cultural heritage and passing down traditions and practices.

- Integrating herbs, plants, and regular rituals can promote balanced well-being and women's health.

- The Divine Feminine is connected to addressing women's health and overall well-being.

- Indigenous cultures have a deep connection to nature and incorporate nature-based practices into self-care routines.

- Honoring and celebrating cultural heritage contributes to holistic well-being.

Your Thoughts Can Make a Difference

Dear Valued Reader,

As our journey together reaches its conclusion, I hope these pages have left an enduring impression on you. Your experience with this book is not just important to me as an author, but it also holds the potential to guide and inspire others.

If you found value in this work, please consider leaving a review on the platform you purchased this book. Your insights and reflections are powerful. They not only help me grow and improve as a writer but also assist others in discovering a book that could enrich their lives as it has yours.

Every review counts, and your voice truly matters in this shared journey of knowledge and discovery.

Thank you for being an integral part of this story, and for considering this request to share your experience with others.

With heartfelt appreciation,

Nya Love

Explore More in the Self Help for Black Women Series

Thank you for spending your time with "African Holistic Health for Women." If this book has inspired and empowered you, you may be delighted to discover more in this series dedicated to the journey of self-help and empowerment for Black women. Each book is a treasure trove of wisdom, tailored to uplift and guide.

1. **Black Women and Narcissists** – Navigate the complex dynamics of relationships with narcissists. This book offers insights and strategies specifically for Black women, empowering you to identify, cope, and thrive beyond these challenging interactions.

2. **Self-Love for Black Women** – A nurturing guide to cultivating self-love and self-care. Explore practices and philosophies that resonate deeply with the unique experiences of Black women, fostering a powerful sense of self-worth and inner peace.

3. **Black Woman Empath** – Discover the strength in sensitivity. This book is a haven for Black women who identify as empaths. Learn how to protect your energy, harness your empathic gifts, and navigate the world with confidence and grace.

4. **Manifesting for Black Women** – Turn dreams into reality. Delve into the art of manifestation, tailored for the unique journey of Black women. Uncover techniques and affirmations that resonate with your spirit and aspirations.

Each book in the series is crafted to resonate with your experiences, challenges, and dreams. Be sure to also check out the accompanying journals available for certain books, such as the Self-Love for Black Women Journal. Continue your journey of self-discovery and empowerment with these transformative reads. You can find Nya Love's complete library by clicking on her name on the platform you purchased this book from to access her author page, or by searching her name.

Awaken Your Inner Goddess: Embrace Your Divine Feminine Energy and Thrive

Have you ever felt a deep longing within you, a yearning to tap into your true power and unleash your inner goddess? Imagine a life where you radiate magnetic confidence, embrace your sensuality, and experience profound self-love and healing. In **"Goddess Energy,"** Kara Lawrence and Nya Love invite you on a transformative journey to connect with your divine feminine energy and reclaim your authentic self.

In this empowering book, Lawrence and Love share their wisdom and insights, guiding you to embrace your femininity and unlock the immense power that lies within you. Drawing on ancient wisdom and modern spirituality, they provide practical techniques and rituals to help you align with your true self, awaken your intuition, and nurture your inner goddess.

- Liberate your hidden potentials and embrace your true power

- Radiate magnetic confidence and attract the life you desire

- Amplify your self-love, sexuality, and sacred healing

- Connect with your sensuality and tap into your intuition

- Cultivate a deeper sense of self-acceptance and body positivity

- Prioritize your well-being and practice self-care rituals

- Discover the transformative power of embracing your emotions

- Embrace your divine feminine energy and live authentically as a modern spiritual being

- Unleash your inner goddess, embrace your divine feminine energy, and embark on a journey of self-discovery and empowerment. Embrace **"Goddess Energy"** and awaken the powerful, radiant woman within you. Find Goddess Energy by Kara Lawrence and Nya Love on ebook, paperback, and audiobook on a variety of platforms.